CLINICAL PEARLS IN REFRACTIVE CARE

CLINICAL PEARLS
IN REFRACTIVE CARE

D. Leonard Werner, O.D., F.A.A.O.

Distinguished Teaching Professor Emeritus, SUNY
State College of Optometry, New York; Regional
Professional Director, Davis Vision, Plainview, New York;
Consultant for Quality Assurance and Professional Staffing,
Vision Clinics, District Council 37, New York

Leonard J. Press, O.D., F.C.O.V.D., F.A.A.O.

Optometric Director, The Vision and Learning Center,
Fair Lawn, New Jersey; Associate Medical Staff, St. Lawrence
Rehabilitation Hospital, St. Lawrence, New Jersey

Foreword by
Jack Runninger, O.D., D.O.S.
Former Editor, *Optometric Management Magazine*

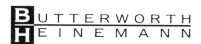

Boston   Oxford   Auckland   Johannesburg   Melbourne   New Delhi

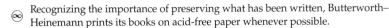
Every effort has been made to ensure that the drug dosage schedules within this text are accurate and conform to standards accepted at time of publication. However, as treatment recommendations vary in the light of continuing research and clinical experience, the reader is advised to verify drug dosage schedules herein with information found on product information sheets. This is especially true in cases of new or infrequently used drugs.

Recognizing the importance of preserving what has been written, Butterworth–Heinemann prints its books on acid-free paper whenever possible.

Library of Congress Cataloging-in-Publication Data

Werner, D. Leonard.
    Clinical pearls in refractive care / D. Leonard Werner, Leonard J. Press; with a foreword by Jack Runninger.
        p. ; cm.
    Includes bibliographical references and index.
    ISBN 0-7506-9912-4 (alk. paper)
    1. Eye—Accommodation and refraction—Case studies. 2. Optometry—Case Studies. I. Press, Leonard J. II. Title.
    [DNLM: 1. Refraction, Ocular. 2. Optometry. WW 300 P935c 2002]
    RE925 .P745 2002
    617.7'5—dc21

                                                                    2001043484

British Library Cataloguing-in-Publication Data

A catalogue record for this book is available from the British Library.

The publisher offers special discounts on bulk orders of this book. For information, please contact:

Manager of Special Sales
Butterworth-Heinemann
225 Wildwood Avenue
Woburn, MA 01801-2041
Tel: 781-904-2500
Fax: 781-904-2620

For information on all Butterworth–Heinemann publications available, contact our World Wide Web home page at: http://www.bh.com

10 9 8 7 6 5 4 3 2 1

Printed in the United States of America

This book is dedicated to our former students and colleagues at the State University of New York's College of Optometry, and to our families who have been supportive of our efforts through the years.

We also acknowledge Karen Oberheim of Butterworth–Heinemann for her encouragement, persistence, and good faith in seeing this project to completion.

Contents

Foreword

"My mother was very resourceful," the late humorist Sam Levenson once reported. He recalled that day when he was a kid and relatives dropped in to visit right at suppertime.

"I'm going to have to invite the relatives to stay for supper, so there won't be enough chicken to go around," Momma told all of us boys. "When the plate is passed around I want you to say that you don't care for any chicken." Even though we were starved we dutifully refused to take any chicken when the food was passed at supper. When everyone had finished Momma announced that she had pie for dessert, but "all you boys who didn't eat your chicken, don't get any pie."

Mrs. Levenson obviously had learned from experience how to come up with commonsense answers to difficult problems. In optometric practice, we also must learn from experience how to come up with commonsense answers, which we term *conventional wisdom*. Optometric care involves more than what we call, in the South, "book larnin'." One of the best ways to learn such conventional wisdom is from mistakes, so we know what to do next time. Even better is learning from the mistakes of others, because we don't live long enough to make all the mistakes ourselves. Or, as the old Pennsylvania Dutch proverb says, "Too soon old, too late smart."

That is why this book by Drs. Werner and Press is so important to the optometric clinician. The commonsense techniques they and other practitioners learned through experience are invaluable to younger practitioners. More experienced practitioners also find methods and thought processes to improve their skills and make them more efficient. The learning of efficient clinical pearls is of even more importance in today's managed care environment. Practitioners must strike a happy balance between time efficiency and good patient care.

"Where are you from?" asked a technician in a major medical clinic as she prepared to take a blood sample from me. "Rome, Georgia," I said happily. At last I had found someone who demonstrated a personal interest in me. All the other technicians had been entirely impersonal. "Are you a native of these parts?" I asked. She proceeded to extract my blood without bothering to answer my question. Then it dawned on me that her inquiry about my hometown was not brought about by any desire to personalize our contact. It was matching the proper record to the blood she was drawing.

I was undergoing a series of tests to determine if I had a tumor. (Fortunately, I did not and have had to search for other excuses for any evidence of stupidity.) There was no eye contact or conversation from any of the testers, except to ask questions for identification purposes. It was a time-efficient method of health care, but it reemphasized to me that patients are people not machines and need to be treated as such.

"How can practitioners demonstrate a caring attitude, garner sufficient examination data to make a good diagnosis, and still operate in a cost-efficient manner?" becomes the important question in today's health care environment. Patient retention and practice enjoyment suffer if clinicians must maintain an assembly-line practice. On the other hand, clinicians who spend too much time with each patient soon go broke if they are accepting reduced fees from managed care. Gone are the days when the optometrist could afford the luxury of spending 45 minutes of face-to-face time with a patient, conducting a 21-point refractive sequence. This book is the first text that addresses this need for balance.

"This instrument measures the curvature of the cornea of your eye and is accurate within 1/200,000 of an inch," I once told a college professor during the course of my examination. I had found that explaining tests I was executing and their results while performing the tests was a "clinical pearl" that helped save time during case presentations. Also I found that patients were impressed by such descriptions. But not this guy! "Obviously that much accuracy is unnecessary," he replied. Too late I realized that, rather than being impressed, he thought I was giving him a snow job. I don't wish to boast, but I am really good at coming up with answers to such rejoinders. In this case the perfect answer I came up with was, "Perhaps not, but I'd rather err on the side of too much accuracy than not enough." The problem was, as always when I come up with good answers, I didn't think of it until 2 hours later, when he was long gone. But the experience showed me that, when you do come up with clinical pearls that are time-savers, you must be certain that they apply specifically to the patient that you're examining.

"It is not the quantity but the quality of time you spend with your patient that is important," I heard Walter Belson, former president of the Public Relations Society of America, once say at an A.O.A. Communications Forum. "Surveys showed that there was no correlation between how well patients thought doctors communicated with them, and the amount of time spent. Many doctors who spend the least time, but used their time well, were judged better communicators than doctors who actually spent much more time with the patient."

The answers to many day-to-day issues are found in this book, which is unique in presenting practical information. To best conceptualize the intent of this text, think of the advice that an experienced clinician would pass on to a new practitioner—the things they don't fully teach you in school about prescribing for patients. The strengths of this text can be summarized as follows:

1. The utilization of automated instrumentation and ancillary personnel.
2. High-yield tests to streamline the refractive process.
3. Steps to utilize in deriving the optimal refractive compensation or correction.
4. The clinical pearls of conventional wisdom in a primary care framework.
5. Identifying common mistakes and pitfalls to be avoided in prescribing lenses.
6. Measures to take when the best laid refractive plans go astray.

It is blatantly apparent that these are important factors for today's practitioner. But the value of any book imparting this knowledge to clinicians depends entirely on the author's knowledge and ability to impart it. The ideal authors for such a text would embody the following qualities.

First, they should be good teachers and have experience in teaching. Drs. Press and Werner were long-time members of the faculty at the State University of New York's College of Optometry. Dr. Werner had such positions as chief of professional services, chair of the department of clinical sciences, and acting dean of the college. Dr. Press served as chief of the vision therapy service and chaired the clinical practice plan. They taught this material at the college within a Case Analysis course for a number of years. They are experienced and respected academicians.

In addition to being good teachers, they should be experienced clinicians who have a grasp of the "real world" of practice. Dr. Press has a full-scope practice in New Jersey and is a well-known authority on vision therapy. Dr. Werner was in private practice and currently is a consultant for quality assurance in managed care programs utilizing record review and monitors many private offices during site visits.

Finally, they should be good writers, who not only know their subject but can explain it in an organized and highly readable manner. When I was editor of *Optometric Management* and later *Optometric Economics*, both Drs. Press and Werner were among my favorite contributors. I found that they always had practical information to impart and did it in an understandable fashion.

Optometric clinicians will find this book and its practical advice to be an invaluable resource that can not only make their practices bigger and better but also more enjoyable.

Jack Runninger, O.D., D.O.S.

Preface

Conventional wisdom (or "pearls") in clinical care are concepts accepted as being true largely because they have been repeated successfully over a long period of time. They have added to their luster from long-time, widespread utilization rather than science, although science has not contradicted their value. Their success and survival add to their acceptance and continued practice. Conventional wisdom has a long history in health care in general and is not idiosyncratic to eyecare. Conventional wisdom is not necessarily dated, and when applied appropriately, it has a role and a place within the contemporary scene.

In the recent past, optometry's concept of a complete examination consisted of a finite list of 21 tests. Completion of these 21 procedures with appropriate interpretation of the relevant data served as a model comprehensive encounter for the bulk of patients. In fact, a basic difference among high-quality practitioners at that time was whether the variation of testing and interpretation was according to one of two principles, graphic analysis or the Optometric Extension Program. With time, many practitioners took what they thought was the best from both philosophies, added others, and the resultant hybrid constituted their full examination and analysis. In some states—New Jersey, for example—the "basic" 21-point examination was written into law, and one did not legally perform a complete ocular examination without completing the 21 steps. As a result of this examination, most patients received a spectacle correction or corrections. This test battery, sometimes with some individual variations, also screened the patient to determine a need for additional testing or referral.

Changes in the scope of optometric practice caused additional tests to be added to this visit. Some of the early examples were biomicroscopy, visual fields, and tonometry. The addition of these procedures had an impact on the scheduled doctor/patient time frame (typically 45 minutes) and some doctors began to selectively eliminate tests, work faster, or delegate. Those patients identified by the testing or history to have other needs (most frequently contact lenses, vision therapy, or suspected ocular disease) were scheduled for additional testing at another visit or referred for outside consultation.

The 21-point basic examination served most patients and, additionally, impressed others who were accustomed to a shorter process. Thus, it had value relating to care, compliance, and practice growth. Frequently, when tests were performed that had a low yield for a specific patient they were rationalized by terming their results *baseline findings*, to be monitored at a later date. It was common to have a specific fee for this basic initial visit. This fee was consistent for all patients regardless of whether an extra test or two was added or eliminated. Interestingly, the same fee usually was charged for monocular and binocular patients, and conversely, the same basic examination was performed regardless of the amount of the fee. It has been likened to "doing the same dance regardless of the music."

Then a new reality came into the picture, the awareness that an additional charge could be generated for an additional procedure. Tonometry was the procedure in optometry that altered the thinking. The invention of the Mackay-Marg tonometer, and later the noncontact tonometer changed the landscape. Politically optometry could no longer be identified by "they do not test for glaucoma." The acquisition of these instruments required an expenditure. The awareness that patients and third parties such as Medicaid would pay additionally for tonometry changed the thinking of many practitioners. Along with the awareness that additional fees can result from additional testing came the expected increased utilization. When the procedure clearly had value in improving care, as was the case with tonometry, the public also benefited. It was the ultimate symbiosis, the patient received better care and the doctor received additional money.

Today we have a very different profession in a changed health care environment. The enlarged scope of optometric practice along with a proliferation of managed care in the form of provider panels, third parties, HMOs, government programs, and varied employment arrangements has changed the economic picture and the professional structure. In many instances, the doctor is not solely in charge of the process or the fee. Those paying the fees indicate what the service is worth and the appropriate frequency for their utilization. Health care (and optometry) is driven by codes and rules, with the likelihood of a test being performed significantly influenced by a reimbursement formula rather than independent professional judgment. The picture is additionally complicated by the capitation system, payment per patient rather than per service, which can dampen the utilization rates of some procedures. Significant changes in professional behavior can be manipulated by the third-party payer, whether a fee for service or capitation concept is employed. The reimbursement concept alters care because with a capitation system increased profit is generated by undertesting and undertreating, while with fee for service overtesting is rewarded. In any third-party system, the solo practitioner with total control of his or her destiny is becoming an endangered species. However, one also must appreciate that, whatever the system of reimbursement, the doctor still has the same professional, moral, and legal responsibility to the patient.

We recognize that much of what we teach must be tempered by the realities of the day. To teach that one must schedule frequent visits prior to making diagnostic and therapeutic closure *usually is not appropriate* in today's streamlined professional world. An example is the scheduling of a separate visit for a cycloplegic evaluation. The self-paying patient may be convinced to accept this as the best approach for his or her specific needs and agree to the fees involved. However, third-party payers may or may not be likely to reimburse for an extended multivisit process. The increased utilization of technology and ancillary personnel encourages the doctor to be more of an analyzer than data gatherer. External forces anticipate that the doctor can arrive at a differential diagnosis with fewer office visits and with less doctor/patient contact time. The absence of authoritative direction in the literature to guide clinicians in this new era gave rise to the need for this book.

Current practice mitigates against each patient having a 45-minute doctor/patient examination encounter for a predetermined 21-point examination at the fee set by the doctor. As the new health system continues to change, a new ocular examination concept is evolving. Patients still have the same set of legitimate expectations for the primary care visit: relief from visual and ocular symptoms and a health screening to rule out the more common and more serious disease processes. Refractively, the doctor still is motivated by a wish to provide visual clarity, comfort, and enhanced binocularity. In addition, when abnormalities are identified, appropriate management strategies need to be employed. This must occur within the time and other constraints created by laws, rules, standards of care, and economics.

While no one can predict the exact dimensions of change that will alter the primary care encounter, we can suggest the conceptual changes that undoubtedly will be necessary to practice at a high level and survive the economic and political pressures. Some doctors already have made some of the necessary changes and they will be best positioned for any eventuality. In this book, we outline the process that will maximize care and caring within a reasonable time frame. Care must be customized for the specific patient with increased utilization of technology and technical assistants and not be a simple lock-step process. In writing this book, we attempt to bridge the gap between theoretical concepts that have shaped eye care and the reality of providing excellent care under different circumstances.

Our goal is to provide the elements that allow for optimum patient care and professional growth. Optimum, not maximum, care will be the standard for most doctors and most patients. This optimum care must still provide for clear, comfortable, efficient vision with the assurance of healthy eyes in a healthy body. It is not our intent for this book to be a reference for secondary or tertiary care. As an example, when contact lenses are a part of the recommended therapy plan, it is not our intention to indicate the type of lens or its parameters. We suggest that the readers review the many fine volumes dedicated to those specific services.

This book evolved from a course we taught, Optometric Case Analysis, in addition to our professional experiences, which span the optometric world from private practice to a multitude of educational, consultative, and administrative activities. It is designed to serve in the real world. This book, like our course, places emphasis on the successful application of "the refraction" terminating in the appropriate spectacle correction. In writing about the refractive process, Duke-Elder and Abrams state, "of all aspects of medicine this practice gives to more people more comfort and increased efficiency than any other medical technique."[1] The appropriate spectacle correction may be the most universally successful medical therapy that exists and the foundation of a successful vision care practice. Satisfying the refractive needs of the patient still forms the backbone of ophthalmic practice growth. In spite of the legal expansion of optometry, the core of eye care practice is refractive care and subsequent spectacle prescriptions.[2] One also should be aware that, as common as refractive care appears to be in our society, unmet needs still may be identified, where refraction can have a significant impact. Tielsch and associates (1995) reported on a study of Baltimore nursing home patients, indicating that 20% of the functional blindness and 37% of the visual impairment found could be rectified by an appropriate refractive correction.[3]

Our contact with professional colleagues makes us aware that some are mired in already outmoded concepts. We recognize a need for this text to serve two different groups: students and recent graduates entering into the current and future health care environment, which may differ from their educational experiences, and practitioners who must contemporize their concepts and practice. Those standing still, in effect, are moving backward.

As clinicians and educators, we are driven by assessment. We typically measure our success with patient or student outcomes. If, as a result of this book, the reader reevaluates the process within his or her professional world and if students and clinical educators consider the implications for them, we have succeeded. Continuing the "old" system will lead to practitioner and patient dissatisfaction.

We try to present a blueprint for care, one that has specificity yet allows for the variation that marks the thoughtful practitioner. New procedures will come of age, old ones may exhibit a rebirth, and most important, outside influences will have an impact on how we deliver care. All these must be subject to the same basic litmus test—whether each is in the best interests of the patient. We must never forget that we are licensed by society to serve the public.

References

1. Duke-Elder S, Abrams D. System of ophthalmology. In: *Ophthalmic Optics and Refraction*, Vol. 5. St. Louis: Mosby, 1970: Preface.
2. Goss DA, Penisten DK. The subordination of refraction. Guest editorial. *J Am Optom Assoc.* October 1996; 67(10): 580–582.
3. Tielsch JM, Javitt JC, Coleman A, Katz B, Sommer A. The prevalence of blindness and visual impairment among nursing home residents in Baltimore. *N Engl J Med.* May 4, 1995; 332(18):1205–1209.

Introduction

"I've taken to the eye, my boy. There's a fortune in the eye. A man grudges a half-crown to cure his chest or his throat, but he'd spend his last dollar over his eye. There's money in ears, but the eye is a gold mine."[1] Times may have changed since the fictional character Cullingworth made this declaration in Sir Arthur Conan Doyle's "The Stark Munro Letters." But it does seem fitting that the author, Conan Doyle, trained in optics and practiced as an eye doctor while creating his most famous fictional character, Sherlock Holmes. After all, in taking relevant clinical history, gathering data, analyzing the information at hand, and formulating a plan, the eye care practitioner functions like a detective.

There is no blueprint for how an individual becomes an efficient detective. Valuable clues that one picks up along the way come from mentors in optometric education, role models in clinical practice, and commonsense advice from esteemed colleagues like Jack Runninger. Dr. Runninger's Foreword should set the tone for the utilization of this book. Widely admired for his ability to express traditional clinical experiences in easy-to-relate-to terms, we endeavor to use this blueprint for style as much as possible.

In both the Foreword and the Preface, the reader will find reference to the impetus that managed care, a particular type of health care system currently rampant in the United States, has given to streamlining clinical care and, in particular, refractive care, even though some practitioners in the eye care marketplace are on the leading edge of a revolution to limit participation in managed care and restore a sense of balance to the doctor/patient relationship. Although we trust that practitioners in managed care environments will find our approach to case analysis and management a useful guide, streamlining data collection and analytical processes should be appealing to all practitioners.

We see at least two other broad applications of discussions about lens prescriptions. The first addresses the concern of influential leaders in our profession who observe that, as our emphasis shifts toward more ostensibly glamorous and valuable disease detection and management skills, we have deemphasized our position as the foremost practitioners of refractive care.[2] An insidious and almost infectious attitude suggests refractive care and other aspects of traditional optometry beyond disease and surgery issues are beneath the dignity of some of our colleagues.[3] If we reduce the growing pains of new practitioners or energize practitioners who find refraction mundane, our efforts will have been rewarded.

The second application we envision revolves around the paradoxes of time. The speeding up and streamlining of processes are not unique to optometric practice. Any decision making that has to be made in "real time" intensifies the concept of nowness.[4] Although virtually unheard of until recently, we now have patients calling our offices on the day of their appointment to ask the receptionist if the doctor is on schedule. There is even clinical folklore about patients sending doctors bills for the time spent waiting to be seen in the doctor's office. Unlike attorneys, optometrists do not bill patients on the basis of the time necessary to inquire about historical data, the time to gather current data based on probes or measures, or conference time applied to differential diagnosis or case presentation. When all these processes, which take time, are not identified to or valued by patients, impatience ensues.

We therefore take the position that, by sharing insights we have gleaned from our own experiences and from input received through colleagues and students over the years, some economy of time can be shared as well. The clinical insights offered are encapsulated in 22 pearls in the opening chapter, "The Pearls of Conventional Wisdom." Although we make numerous references to these pearls (by number and in bold type) in later chapters, we also interject other perils and pearls of clinical refractive judgment when appropriate.

After setting the tone for our book in the first chapter, we progress to the topic of autorefraction. This new technology has been positioned as another opportunity to delegate procedures, save time, and increase patient flow.[5] However, it also begs the question of what is meant by *refraction* and the responsibilities of a refractionist. Guidelines published by the American Optometric Association support a restricted view of refraction as a determination of the lens prescription needed to provide optimal visual acuity for all viewing distances.[6] Other aspects of the examination, such as entering visual acuity, lensometry, cover test, near point of convergence (NPC), accommodative amplitude, and stereopsis, are distinct from the refraction.

Through case examples, we demonstrate when autorefraction can be used as a stand-alone process. In doing so, we are mindful of the aphorism attributed to Albert Einstein, to make things as simple as possible, but not simpler.[7] This point often is obscured or trivialized by the debate over what delegation of this technology signifies. Synthesizing the data gathered and formulating lens prescriptions best suited to the patient's needs will always remain within the province of the doctor. Far more than bells and whistles, integrated autorefraction is deceptively elegant and streamlines the refractive process. Its intelligent application is by no means simple.

The bulk of the chapters in this text incorporates a template intended to make it simpler for the reader to follow our clinical lines of thought. The template has the following structure:

Subjective
Case history, including signs, symptoms, and visual needs
Lensometry
Objective
Ocular health assessment
Clinical measures:
At 20 ft (6 m)
At 16 in. (40 cm)
VA (cc):
OD
OS

Cover test
N.P.C.
Retinoscopy/autorefractor
Subjective:
OD   VA
OS   VA
Phoria:
    Base-in vergences
    Base-out vergences
Accom. amplitude
Neg. rel. accom.
Pos. rel. accom.
Fused X-cyl.
Stereo
Assessment
Plan

In working through the various case examples, the reader will encounter *N/E* as a notation after some of the clinical findings, to indicate that the data were *not essential* to clinical decision making. Little justification can be found for collecting data if the doctor has no intention of using such data in making a decision. There are rare exceptions, as when the practitioner is a provider for a third-party vision plan that dictates the minimum database required. In any event, we are mindful that, in specific cases, you may not agree with our choices as to which data are essential to the derivation of a lens prescription.

As you proceed through these chapters, bear in mind that each case involves patient encounters in which the authors were directly involved. They are not composites or theoretically illustrative cases. In caring for a wide variety of patients, we had the luxury of selecting cases that reflect good decisions as well as mistakes we made. As long as you practice optometry, you continue to learn. Each case brings alternatives and options, which we elaborate. When applicable, we refer to the clinical pearls from Chapter 1 and the correlates that guided our decisions. We trust that they will illuminate your clinical refractive pathways.

References

1. Booth M. *The Doctor and the Detective: A Biography of Sir Arthur Conan Doyle.* New York: Thomas Dunne Books, 2000: 119.
2. Borish IM, Catania LJ. Putting optics back into primary care. *Optom Management.* 1998;33(10):22–28.
3. Runninger J. I don't fool with glasses. *Optom Management.* 1998;33(10):14.
4. Gleick J. *Faster: The Acceleration of Just about Everything.* New York: Pantheon Books, 1999:67.
5. Buscemi PM. A new approach to refraction. *Optom Management.* 1999;34(3):40.
6. *Comprehensive Adult Eye and Vision Examination: Reference Guidelines for Clinicians.* St. Louis: American Optometric Association, 1994.
7. Nichols R. Opening remarks: Unity of knowledge—The convergence of natural and human science. *Annals of the New York Academy of Sciences.* 2001;935:x (Introduction).

CHAPTER 1

The Pearls of Conventional Wisdom

When one speaks of the art and science of health care it is the essential melding of practicality of what works with the scientific rationale. We traditionally refer to these practically acquired guidelines that prevail through time as *conventional wisdom*, but the contemporary professional literature calls them *pearls*. In developing a list of such pearls, a group of faculty, both optometrists and ophthalmologists, were asked to submit the rules that have best served them through the years. There were many redundancies. Milder and Rubin, in their text, also identify some rules and, not surprisingly, some of these appeared on our unofficial list.[1] Due to the nature of such a list, contributors have suggested items reported elsewhere. The lack of references reflects the acceptance of these as a part of the public domain rather than any attempt to suggest authorship to other's gems. These pearls will reappear when they apply to specific cases elsewhere in the book. Some of these pearls follow, in no particular order.

Pearl 1: Listen to Your Patient

Your patient will tell you what is wrong and, sometimes, how to correct it. Using open-ended questions and allowing the patient time to respond, while observing his or her body language, present the clinician with a great deal of information. For example, the myopic patient who reports poor distance vision with her glasses that she can improve by tilting her spectacles to be closer

1

to her eyes clearly indicates that an increase in minus lens power improves her distance vision. Tilting to allow the lower portion of the lenses to be closer to the eye increases the effective power of the minus spectacle lens. The presbyopic patient who pushes his plus lenses further down his nose is increasing their effective power and telling the practitioner that he may prefer to see at near with stronger plus lenses.

Pearl 2: Sensitive Patients Require Very Precise Prescriptions (Others Need Only Exact Ones)

We learn about this heightened sensitivity by the patient's subjective responses during the testing sequence as well as remarks made during the case history. For example, the patient who reports poor distance vision and misses only one letter on the 20/15 (6/4.5) line may be an example of this, particularly when she responds with confidence in discerning small lens changes while being subjectively examined. This patient often reacts with confidence to small incremental differences during the Jackson cross-cylinder test. She also shows a heightened reaction when her glasses are poorly fabricated, ill-fitting, or dirty.

Pearl 3: Myopes Have a Right to Their Seeing Preferences

Patients may want their sight to be fully corrected or undercorrected. The reduced acuity goal for the myopic patient usually can be traced to the "theory" that one should undercorrect a myope to prevent progression of the myopia. As a therapy designed to either reduce the myopia or prevent its progression, undercorrection has been controversial. Undoubtedly, a group of myopic patients do not see as well as they might or ought to. However, the myopic individual who subjectively prefers to see things "softer" or slightly blurred has a right to his preference. The ethicist refers to this as patient autonomy. Whether this preference is to actually reduce the sharpness in their visual world or a subconscious effort of reducing their perceived degree of myopia (or the thickness of the correcting lenses), the clinician's role is to present the options to the patient along with recommendations. If the patient's preference differs from the clinician's and is not harmful, this should be respected. One need not be dogmatic about the absolute value of 0.25 diopters.

Pearl 4: Use Trial Lenses with Every Significant Lens Change

If you do not know if the change is significant, use trial lenses. If the tentative change is for distance seeing, allow the patient to walk around with this prescription. If there is a window nearby, allow the patient to view distant signs or scenery. Slight distance blur is more easily observed by the patient if asked to view detail at a distance. This distance should be greater than the length of the examination room.

Pearl 5: Be Very Cautious About Reducing Minus at Distance with the Myopic Patient or (5A) Reducing the Net Plus Power at Near with a Presbyopic Patient

Some of our respondents used the word *never* instead of suggesting caution when considering these changes. Under certain conditions, one might circumvent either of these rules but only with the doctor and the patient fully understanding the implications of this approach.

Some students forget that both prescriptions A and B in the following example have the same total net plus power at near and that C represents a significant increase in the total net plus power at near:

A. OU: +2.00 DS/+2.00 add
B. OU: +3.00 DS/+1.00 add
C. OU: +3.00 DS/+2.00 add

Pearl 6: Be Cautious in Making Asymmetrical Prescription Changes

One should consider that this type of change is significant and apply pearl 4, the use of trial lenses. The asymmetry may relate to power or axis changes that are different for one eye than the other or equal in power but dissimilar axis changes. This pearl can have implications at distance or near.

Pearl 7: Never Prescribe More Plus Power at Distance Than Is Consistent with Good Distance Vision

A rare exception to this is when there is good reason to believe that the "true" refractive error, as might be revealed with cycloplegia, results in more plus power in the correction than the patient seems to accept subjectively without cycloplegia. Another example is when this added plus power improves fusion with a patient having an eso deviation. If you decide to prescribe accordingly, do it with extreme caution and full patient understanding. Some suggest that it should be attempted along with, or following, a "plus acceptance" process, such as vision therapy, or preceding the distance application with additional plus power for near.

A common cause of dissatisfaction is vision that is slightly blurred at distance because of too much plus lens power at far. The amount of power that can generate the unhappiness can be as little as 0.25 or 0.50 diopters. Strangely, undercorrected myopic patients are less likely to present this symptom than patients with a hyperopic component, perhaps because myopic patients have become accustomed to distance blur. Several methods can be employed to guard against too much distance plus power. Some practitioners apply the "green rule" in the red/green bichrome test. This has been expressed jokingly as, "keep them [patients] in the green and they'll keep you in the green." Another approach is to not prescribe more distance plus than was uncovered with static "dry" retinoscopy. A third process is the +1.00 check test. Placing +1.00 sphere over the tentative distance correction should blur the patient to approximately 20/60 (6/18) visual acuity. If the acuity is poorer than that, beware of too much distance plus in the tentative prescription. If the acuity is better, be aware of the possibility of not enough distance plus power.

The best way to guard against causing distance blur is to place the tentative prescription in the trial frame and ask the patient to view a distant target beyond the confines of the examination room.

Pearl 8: It Often Is Prudent in Making a Lens Change of 1 Diopter or More to Prescribe It in Stages

If, however, you choose to consider a lens change of this magnitude, consider using trial lenses before prescribing. Changes of this magnitude may have implications at far or near. As an example, increasing the prescription of a young myopic patient by −1.50 requires the patient to accommodate 1.50 diopters more at near than before the lens change, with a subsequent alteration in the binocularity. If making a change of this amount, inform the patient that, along with increased distance clarity, he or she may notice that things initially seem different when reading or doing near seeing. Moderation in change is called for when the AC/A ratio is high.

Pearl 9: In General, a Lens Change of Less Than 0.50 Diopters Seldom Diminishes Subjective Asthenopic Symptoms

One exception might be a very sensitive presbyopic patient who can appreciate that an increase of +0.25 at near improves near vision or an equally sensitive myopic patient who might appreciate increased clarity with the change of −0.25 at distance, but these patients are the exceptions to the rule. Also, we cannot quantify the degree of subjective reaction by a patient knowing a change is being made, however small. If you make a change of this 0.25 amount, be cautious in what you suggest as to its benefit. If the patient is advised that a 0.25 power change in one eye will eliminate his frequent headaches, he will either be misled or you succeeded with a placebo therapy. However, the use of trial lenses might generate the clarity responses to help with the decision.

A number of studies demonstrate that repetitive refractive findings are overwhelmingly within 0.50 diopters of each other, attesting to the repeatability of the testing process. As a result, one can state that, if a difference of 0.50 diopters or more is found, it probably represents a change in refractive status and is worthy of consideration.[2]

Pearl 10: Never Modify the Cylindrical Power Without Considering Its Effect on the Spherical Component

A carefully measured binocular balance and its resultant acuity may be lost by modifying the cylindrical lens prescription lens without considering the spherical equivalent. For example, as a result of the distance binocular subjective examination that, by definition, equalizes the accommodative levels of the two eyes, we find

OD: +2.00 –2.00 × 90   VA 20/20 (6/6)
OS: +1.75 –0.75 × 90   VA 20/20 (6/6)

If the patient presented wearing a –1.00 cylinder in the OD, when we place this prescription in a trial frame, it causes the patient to report space distortion. Reducing the cylinder of the OD to –1.50 eliminates this distortion. To compensate for the effect on the sphere, the lenses for the OD should be +1.75 –1.50 × 90. The distance acuity of the OD should be measured again with this new combination—it probably will approximate 20/20 (6/6), although it is always a good idea to measure so that you have this finding for the prescribed lens. Simply eliminating some of the cylinder and keeping the +2.00 OS for the right lens will reduce acuity and alter the binocular accommodative balance.

Pearl 11: Never Prescribe Without Understanding the Patient's Visual Needs (and Seeing Distances) and Appreciating the Effect of the New Prescription on These Needs (and Distances)

You must ask about these needs during the case history and note the answers on the record. The effect of increasing the minus power at distance with a pre-presbyopic myopic patient may illustrate this. Additional minus power at distance reduces the overall plus at near and may generate near symptoms with a patient having reduced accommodation. Undercorrected myopic spectacle-wearing patients between 35 and 40 years of age who became fully corrected with either contact lenses or refractive surgery now present with symptoms of early presbyopia.

Pearl 12: Be Careful in Changing the Lens Design with High Prescriptions

Anything above 3 diopters could be considered high. The lens clock should be applied *and curves noted* when the previous prescription is neutralized. In addition, a notation should be made of the distance between optical centers, lens material, lens thickness, multifocal type, tint, and the like. If the patient is asymptomatic, if possible, all aspects of the previous prescription, including the distance between optical centers, should be duplicated.

Pearl 13: There Is No Rule Limiting the Near Add to +2.50

Many practitioners have had great success with patients who required more than a +2.50 addition, some of them have attained the title *low-vision specialist*. The most successful low-vision aid is a high near add (see Chapter 12).

Pearl 14: Follow the Generic Therapeutic Rules

The generic therapeutic rules have stood the test of time in all of the health professions. Some of these are

It is difficult to improve on an asymptomatic state.
If it ain't broke, don't fix it.
If it is working keep doing it, and the opposite approach, if it isn't working stop doing it.
Above all do no harm.

In spite of being aware of these, many practitioners have patients returning with complaints because, in a moment of weakness (or elevated self-worth), they neglected these rules. We must caution the reader that we define *asymptomatic* by more than subjectivity. Clearly, the patient with open-angle glaucoma but no subjective symptoms does not meet the standard of being asymptomatic nor the nonachieving child with binocular deficits who does not report asthenopic symptoms.

Pearl 15: The Patient's Last Doctor May Have Been Wiser Than You Initially Thought

The doctor may not have missed something you uncovered, but she may have wisely chosen not to act on it, so there may have been good reasons for her decision. Some examples of this are

1. Intentionally creating a monovision correction to increase the range of clarity at near with a presbyopic patient.
2. Undercorrecting a cylinder.
3. Modifying a cylinder axis to be less oblique.

In developing this list of pearls, some of the other contributions listed provide valuable guidance to the practitioner. Some of these have practice management significance, patient confidence implications, or encourage compliance; others may have practical value. As a result we add the following pearls.

Pearl 16: Exert Care in Telling the Patient What Benefits to Expect from the New Prescription

Patients become unhappy when their expectations are not realized. These expectations sometimes are revealed to sensitive practitioners during the case history. The clinician who explains any possible shortcomings or side effects of the new correction may avoid future problems. All these should be repeated when the glasses are dispensed. The limitations of a single-vision near-lens prescription on an early presbyope cannot be overemphasized. Demonstrate to the patient that he is unable to see well at a distance with this approach. Some patients think that reading road signs or movie titles is what we mean by reading. We find that a better descriptive term is *near-seeing glasses*, with a demonstration of their effective seeing range. The patient receiving his first single-vision near correction understands when told that these glasses are for seeing things sufficiently close to be hand held.

Pearl 17: The Patient Should Understand the Prognosis of His or Her Eye Condition

The young myope may get worse and the early presbyope will get worse and, unless something else intervenes (such as refractive surgery, injury, or pathology), both most likely will continue to need corrective eyewear in the future, regardless of whether they comply in wearing their glasses. We all have heard disappointed presbyopic patients complain that their wearing of a prescription at near resulted in the inability to read without them several years later.

Pearl 18: Remind All Patients That They May Have to Adapt to Their New Glasses

This applies even if the new glasses duplicate the previous spectacles. Many eyeglass-wearing patients have experienced discomfort or space distortion in the past with new glasses so this subtly reinforces what they might experience. Using this approach results in a win/win situation because, if some patient adjustment is necessary, it is no surprise; if not, they will be pleased how easily they adapted and might credit you with this success. *Apply this pearl liberally.*

Pearl 19: Avoid Examining Close Relatives, Refer Them to Distant Colleagues

This requires little elaboration. The first "failure" for one of us was his father. He ignored pearls 4, 5, 6, 14, 15, and 18, as well as 19. The patient did not appreciate the off-axis cylinders in both eyes after never having worn them and presenting with no symptoms—particularly after those heavy tuition bills.

Pearl 20: If the Patient Presents with a Shopping Bag Full of Unsatisfactory Spectacles, You Probably Will Add to the Collection

In spite of this caution, it is incumbent on you to try to help. Perhaps the combination of your skill, timing, knowledge, and charisma will prevail. There is great satisfaction in helping patients in this category, however rare. In these situations pearl 18 also applies.

Pearl 21: When We Perform Clinical Measures at Near and Interpret the Results, Remember That Few People Read at Eye Level with the Material Suspended from a Near-Point Rod

A notable exception to this, at least relating to the angle of sight, is the computer screen. The near-point rod allows us to simulate the computer screen distance (and sometimes location), if needed, but not the typical reading posture.

Pearl 22: Balanced Accommodative (and Focal) Levels Help Ensure Happy Patients

If at all possible, prescribe lenses that equalize the accommodative or near focal levels of the two eyes of the patient. This is more important than equalizing the near acuities. (An example of this may be found in the Chapter 13, relating to dissatisfied patients.) We discussed equal accommodative levels with pearl 10, as it related to the distance prescription, it also applies at near. If your testing suggests the need for unequal adds (and sometimes they are necessary), first recheck the accommodative balance at distance. A method to determine the potential need for unequal adds is to perform monocular ranges through the tentative near prescription. In this way, we can measure the accommodative amplitude and learn if the prescription meets the near distance needs of the patient. An important exception to this occurs when an asymptomatic patient has acquired or induced variations of monovision.

If you follow these rules you will have success as a refractionist. However, the excellent clinician understands that rules can be broken when appropriate.

References

1. Milder B, Rubin ML. *The Fine Art of Prescribing Glasses*, Vol. 2. Gainesville, FL: Triad Publishing Company, 1991:3, 4.
2. Goss DA, Grosvenor T. Reliability of refraction—A literature review. *J Am Optom Assoc.* October 1996;67(10):619–630.

CHAPTER 2

Autorefractor Applications to Lens Prescribing

Two optometrists were overheard at a practice management meeting discussing their latest strategies. When one complained about stagnation in the growth of his practice, the other replied: "Why don't you do what I did? Convince the ophthalmologist down the road to buy an autorefractor." Rubin and Milder, anticipating possible overreliance on the delegation of refraction and its impact on the lens prescriptions, noted the following:

> But, you may wonder, are good refractionists in danger of becoming superfluous? Will the need for the clinician's skills be usurped by those new, remarkable, sophisticated refraction machines? Absolutely not! There will always be a demand for the expertise of the refracting clinician who can satisfy a patient's needs and who, by applying common sense, can translate even objectively-derived refraction findings in to subjectively pleasing corrective prescriptions.[1]

Our aim in this chapter is to contribute to commonsense approaches that help formulate a satisfactory lens prescription from objectively derived autorefractive findings. An automated refractor is an instrument that determines the refractive state of the eye by monitoring the retinal image rather than requiring interpretation of the image by a clinician.[2] The modern concept of automated refraction probably can be traced to Aaron Safir's ophthalmetron, in effect an automated retinoscope, introduced in 1972.[3] In general, the literature has produced favorable reports of the accuracy of automated refractors.[4,5] The traditional retinoscope remains a

13

better tool when the patient has small pupils or media disturbances and with some patients after refractive surgery procedures.[6]
As will be discussed later in this chapter, the instrument environment of autorefractors may overstimulate accommodation, resulting in pseudomyopia.[7]

The concept of automation-assisted refraction has generated
considerable discussion in recent years.[8] The bulk of attention in
such discussions often is directed toward a debate about the relative merits of delegating refraction.[9,10] Elwin Marg, one of optometry's pioneers in computer-assisted practice, envisions the most
important contribution of automation to eye examination to be
economic.[11] We would like to redirect the spotlight from economics
toward the technology itself and specifically the extent to which
autorefractors can provide the clinician insight beyond what traditionally is obtained by manual refraction. Not wishing to side-
step the issue of delegating refraction, we include perspectives on
this aspect of automated refraction at the end of the chapter.

A variety of autorefactors are available commercially. Although we center the discussion on the one with which we have
the most clinical experience, the same principles apply to other
autorefraction systems. The unit we use is the Nidek autorefractor,[12] and we highlight several component features. The Nidek
autorefractor is linked to an autophoropter, and we discuss some
advantages to this linkage later in this chapter.

First, think of autorefraction as computerized retinoscopy.
We refer to the autorefractor as a *smart retinoscope*, but you have to
learn how to interpret its results intelligently. Clearly, autorefraction allows you to delegate the objective refraction, but making
full use of the unique contributions of current units goes well
beyond automated retinoscopy. Retinoscopy is a learned art, and
under some conditions, the interpretation of the retinoscopic reflex requires clinical judgment. Examples include scissors motion
as observed in keratoconus, brightness changes as observed in
accommodative spasm or infacility, and obstruction of the reflex
observed with lenticular opacification. Autorefractor findings
need not necessarily replace retinoscopy but might alert the practitioner for the need to conduct supplemental retinoscopy. This
certainly is the case when objective information is desired about

near-point focusing, which requires the examiner to conduct near-point retinoscopy. We therefore take the position that it is possible to use an autorefractor as a primary objective tool for refraction and reserve the retinoscope for confirmatory or supplemental findings.

After gaining some experience with the features of automated refractors, the practitioner can quantify variables that otherwise would be qualitative. For example, it has been suggested that dulling of the normal bright-red reflex color reflects a relative inattention to the fixation target at near.[13] The same principle applies when the patient is asked to fixate the distance target. Any factor that interferes with accurate fixation or the state of accommodation may result in variability of each autorefractor reading, low confidence values for each reading, or some combination of both, as discussed in the next section.

Variables in Autorefractor Findings

Anything affecting the stability or quality of the light reflex pathway in or out of the eye is a potential source of variability in autorefraction. In short, whatever serves as a source of fluctuation in retinoscopic reflexes also causes fluctuation in autorefractor findings. Most autorefractors allow the practitioner to preselect how many spherocylindrical readings will be taken. The number of readings can be as many as five, but standard practice is three findings for each eye. As we demonstrate, looking at the extent of agreement between the three findings is significant. Table 2-1 lists a number of potential sources of variability, although our main focus will be on accommodation.

When obtaining findings with most autorefractors, the patient is directed to look at a target designed to minimize accommodation. For example, Rodenstock's CX-520 has a sailboat on the ocean. Topcon's 8000PA has a barn at the end of a long farm road. Nidek's ARK 700 has a hot air balloon in the sky at the end of a highway. Irrespective of the target and an internal autofogging procedure, the patient's awareness of looking inside the peephole of an instrument is likely to introduce some instrument myopia. Other than cycloplegia, the most effective way to minimize overaccommodation is to

Table 2-1   Sources of Variability in Autorefraction

Eyelids: Long eyelashes, ptosis
Unstable precorneal tear film
Keratoconus
Refractive surgery
Media opacities (cornea or lens)
Small or irregular pupils
Accommodative spasm
Amblyopia
Poor fixation

use an autorefactor that provides an open, binocular view. Grand Seiko's WR-5100K is unique in allowing the patient to view an external target across the room while conducting autorefraction. The open view unit also has a near-point rod, which permits objective autorefraction at 40 cm or any distance desired.

The autorefractor that we use primarily, Nidek's ARK-700A, typically takes three readings of each eye. In addition to displaying the sphere, cylinder, and axis for each reading, the printout of the findings shows a confidence value for each reading, with the lowest value typically at 5 and the highest value at 9. Use of the confidence interval is a key element in the intelligent interpretation of autorefractive data. If the light reflex that the autorefractor is neutralizing is bright and stable, the reading should be rated 9. If there is interference with or instability in the light path, the reading obtained will be less than 9 and can be as low as 5. If the image quality is poor enough to register less than 5, the confidence factor will be displayed as E, or error. Each reading includes the sphere, cylinder, and axis and is followed on the printout by a suggested best fit of the data based on the three readings.

It is best to conceptualize the internal consistency of the findings as an index of repeatability and the confidence value as an index of reliability. However, as we show, variability between measures or low confidence values do not always mean that the data are invalid or unreliable. Rather, often the explanation for the variance might provide important diagnostic clues. Although it is valid to use the averaged or best-fit reading as a starting point for the subjective refraction, it is important to look at the internal consistency of the three readings. To illustrate, we display the confidence factor in parentheses and the best-fit data in brackets. For ease of discussion, we refer to the spherocylindrical best-fit data as the *outcome value*. Consider the following example:

–0.50 –1.00 × 90 (9)
–0.50 –1.25 × 90 (9)
–0.50 –1.00 × 89 (9)
Outcome value: [–0.50 –1.00 × 90]

In this case, all three readings are in good agreement, and each has a high confidence value (9). The outcome value, –0.50 –1.00 × 90, is a reasonable starting point for the subjective refraction and should be close to the final value obtained in most cases. Contrast this with the following set of readings:

–0.75 –1.75 × 105 (7)
–1.00 –1.00 × 70 (8)
+0.25 –0.50 × 80 (8)
Outcome value: [–0.50 –1.00 × 80]

In this case, the three readings are not in agreement, and each falls short of the optimal confidence value (9). The outcome value, –0.50 –1.00 × 80, is a reasonable starting point for the subjective refraction, but we lack a high degree of confidence that this value will provide the best acuity or be the prescription given.

We have used the autorefractor as objective autoretinoscopy for children as young as 3 years of age. The internal target of the Nidek Autorefractor (ARK-700), a hot air balloon in the sky hovering over a highway, generally is an effective stimulus in maintaining and simulating distance fixation. But this is not always the case, and there is a tendency for autorefractors with internal fixation targets to overminus patients. When beginning the subjective refraction of a young patient, we tend to reduce the autorefractor finding by at least –0.50 sph as a starting point. A clue to how much the autorefractor is overminusing the patient can be gained by noting the patient's unaided acuity or aided acuity through the habitual lens prescription. For example, if an asymptomatic patient is wearing –3.00 sph OU that provides 20/20 visual acuity and the autorefractor findings are –4.00 sph OU, the patient is likely overaccommodating to the stimulus by 1 diopter.

Therefore, when the patient is less than 45 years old and the internal consistency of the three readings is poor, think first of accommodative fluctuation as the source of variability. This may be true even when the confidence value is high for each of the three readings. Since accommodative excess or pseudomyopic responses may be highly labile, the autoretinoscopy feature of autorefractors is unique in its ability provide dynamic, real-time data. This is true not only of significant variability in sphere value but in cylindrical value and axis orientation as well. Although an experienced retinoscopist might use brightness and other cues to detect fluctuation, it is difficult if not impossible to quantify the extent of variability that some patients exhibit. We therefore propose that, in detecting distance refractive fluctuation secondary to accommodative instability, the autorefractor offers unique insight and documentation. Reviewing the internal consistency of the readings, the confidence intervals, and any differences between left eye and right eye facilitates explanation of the condition to patients or parents.

We also use the autorefractor as an objective tool to document the difference between manifest and cycloplegic refractions attributable to accommodative excess or latent hyperopia. Typically, the cycloplegic findings will show not only less myopia but increased internal consistency between readings and higher confidence values. Amblyopia is another cause of internal inconsistency in autorefractor readings. In that event, the confidence value probably will be less than 9 for one or more of the readings obtained through the amblyopic eye. This will be in contrast with the internal consistency and high confidence values obtained through the nonamblyopic eye.

Confidence values less than 9 obtained during auotrefraction of senior citizens usually are associated with lenticular changes. Disturbances in the media make it hard to obtain consistent readings. The confidence value tends to decrease in direct proportion to the density of the cataract. In our clinical experience, when the confidence value falls below 8, the likelihood is that the best-corrected visual acuity is less than 20/25 and the patient is coping with reduced visual function. Aside from contrast sensitivity testing, we find the confidence value of autorefraction valuable in counseling the patient about the advisability of cataract surgery. Particularly for returning patients, a reduction in the confidence value provides an objective index of reduced image quality.

When readings become difficult to obtain due to a patient's long eyelashes, the examiner can manually raise the eyelid. If poor readings are attributable to small pupil size, dimming the room illumination may be of assistance. When poor fixation accounts for errors in the reading, the autorefractor can be switched to the manual mode. This allows the examiner to encourage the patient's fixation and to depress the trigger button only when the patient's eye is centered, as viewed through the monitor on the examiner's side.

Case Examples

Subjective

Case History, Including Signs, Symptoms, and Visual Needs

HB, a 36-year-old administrative assistant, has no previous lens prescription and her chief complaint is that distance signs are difficult to read when driving, particularly at night. Glare from oncoming headlights is not a significant problem as compared with reading signs. Unaided distance acuity is 20/30 (6/9) in each eye. Manifest autorefractor findings are as follows:

OD: −1.50 −0.25 × 41 (9)
       −2.00 −0.00 × 0 (9)
       −2.00 −0.25 × 32 (9)
OS: −1.50 −0.50 × 68 (9)
       −1.75 −0.25 × 69 (9)
       −1.50 −0.25 × 155 (9)

Subjective refraction is −0.50 sphere OU, which affords 20/20 (6/6) acuity at distance. Based on trial lens acuity and responses, we prescribe –0.50 sph OU to be used primarily when driving. HB's autorefraction shows excessive minus lens power, most likely due to accommodative excess. In this case, other refractive findings or near-point analyses are not essential in deriving the lens prescription. Although optometric vision therapy might be an option to lessen HB's pseuodmyopia, she claims to have neither the time nor resources to pursue vision therapy.

Subjective

Case History, Including Signs, Symptoms, and Visual Needs

AM is an 11-year-old child for whom we previously prescribed single-vision lenses of +0.50 sphere OU to be used for near activities. She reports that her vision occasionally is blurry and admits that she has not been using her glasses. She is not certain if blur is more noticeable at distance or near and does not remember if the blur occurs more with one eye than the other. Her unaided visual acuity is 20/20 (6/6) at distance and near without correction. AM's manifest autorefractor findings are as follows:

OD: +0.00 –0.00 × 0 (9)
       –2.00 –0.25 × 174 (9)
       –1.25 –0.25 × 155 (9)
OS: +0.00 –0.00 × 0 (9)
       +0.00 –0.00 × 0 (9)
       +0.00 –0.00 × 0 (9)

Given the high confidence factors, it is evident that AM is exhibiting a variable pseudomyopia of the right eye, in contrast with stable refraction of the left eye. Our advice is that AM should use her near-point prescription more often and that we expect this to stabilize her visual acuity.

Subjective

Case History, Including Signs, Symptoms, and Visual Needs

EB is a 47-year-old school secretary with an ocular history significant for periodic iritis. Her last episode was 2 years ago, treated by an ophthalmologist in a nearby town. EB occasionally experiences glare and dull pain in the left eye, both of which have been chronic complaints. EB experiences some variability in her vision and formerly had been unable to adapt to multifocal lenses. She is interested in new frames and wants to try a multifocal lens again. Her unaided distance visual acuity is 20/25 +1 (6/7.5 +1) OD and 20/20 −1 (6/6 −1) OS. Visual acuity at near through her current reading glasses is 20/20 −2 (6/6 −2) with either eye. The lensometry of her single-vision reading prescription is

OD: +2.25 −0.50 × 165
OS: +1.50 −0.50 × 160

Her intraocular pressures are 15 mm OD and 14 mm OS; all other eye health findings are normal except for mild chemosis and trace cells and flare in the anterior chambers of both eyes.

EB's manifest autorefractor findings are as follows:

OD: −0.25 −1.00 × 101 (6)
    +0.00 −1.25 × 112 (6)
    −0.25 −1.00 × 113 (6)
OS: −0.75 −0.75 × 90 (7)
    −0.50 −1.00 × 93 (7)
    −0.50 −1.00 × 94 (7)

Suspecting that she has a low-grade recurrence of iritis and this may have some impact on her accommodation, we instill 1% cyclopentolate, and the cycloplegic autorefractor findings are as follows:

OD: +1.00 −0.75 × 106 (8)
    +0.75 −0.50 × 100 (8)
    +1.00 −0.75 × 101 (7)
OS: +0.50 −0.50 × 96 (8)
    +0.50 −0.50 × 94 (8)
    +0.50 −0.50 × 98 (8)

Note the discrepancy in cylinder axis between EB's habitual prescription and her current refraction. We counsel EB on the source of variability in her vision and suggest that, although we feel a multifocal lens would be beneficial, we would wait until a short course of mild, topical cycloplegia and steroid application quieted her anterior chamber inflammation. EB returns 10 days later, and her manifest autorefractor findings are as follows:

OD: +0.75 –0.75 × 163 (9)
    +0.75 –0.75 × 163 (9)
    +0.75 –0.75 × 165 (9)
OS: +0.75 –0.75 × 167 (9)
    +0.50 –0.50 × 168 (9)
    +0.50 –0.50 × 167 (9)

Note the improved internal consistency of the findings in each eye, as well as the increase in respective confidence values. Subjective refraction, providing 20/20 (6/6) acuity in each eye, is as follows:

OD: +0.75 –0.75 × 163
OS: +0.50 –0.50 × 167

We prescribe 0.25 less plus sphere than the distance refraction and, based on the near-point findings, derive the following progressive addition lens prescription:

OD: +0.25 –0.75 × 163/+2.25
OS: +0.25 –0.50 × 167/+2.25

We reduce the plus at distance to avoid overplussing EB at distance, yet still provide some improvement compared to unaided distance acuity. Given her history, there is a good chance that she will continue to undergo periodic episodes of iritis of varying intensity. For those times when she needs more distance plus power, she can elevate her chin slightly to obtain more plus power through the upper region of the intermediate lens area. Had we prescribed full plus for distance and EB experienced some spasm, she would be obliged to remove her glasses.

Subjective

Case History, Including Signs, Symptoms, and Visual Needs

Sometimes the autorefractor is helpful in deciding what not to prescribe. JL is a 9-year-old child who is large physically for his age but quite immature emotionally. He struggles to earn passing grades at school, which seems at odds with his verbal abilities. JL has no complaints about his clarity at distance or near, although his parents report that he likes to get close to the page when reading. Unaided visual acuities at distance and near are 20/25 (6/7.5) and manifest autorefractor readings are as follows:

OD: Plano –0.50 × 166 (9)
    –0.25 –0.50 × 180 (9)
    –0.25 –0.50 × 169 (9)
OS: –5.50 –1.25 × 24 (6)
    –8.25 –1.00 × 4 (9)
    –8.00 –1.00 × 172 (7)

The findings point toward a powerful pseudomyopic response of the left eye. After conducting other tests, which produce nebulous responses, we repeat the manifest autorefraction and obtain the following results:

OD: –9.75 –1.00 × 176 (7)
    –10.00 –1.50 × 180 (6)
    –10.00 –1.25 × 6 (7)
OS: –7.25 –1.50 × 8 (7)
    –8.25 –1.50 × 179 (E)
    –2.00 –1.75 × 177 (E)
    –1.75 –0.75 × 175 (9)
    –7.25 –1.25 × 174 (8)

It seems clear that JL has a highly variable pseudomyopia, including astigmatic variabilities. We therefore are interested in documenting what would happen in a more relaxed accommodative state. We cycloplege JL with 1% cyclopentolate and obtain the following autorefractor findings:

OD: −0.50 −0.25 × 128 (9)
    −2.75 −1.25 × 10 (8)
    −3.50 −1.75 × 6 (6)
OS: −5.25 −2.75 × 169 (E)
    −2.75 −1.25 × 179 (9)
    −2.00 −1.00 × 173 (9)

Since JL has reasonably good acuity for his age at distance and near, prescribing a minus lens prescription that might enable JL to identify one or two additional letters on the Snellen chart would be counterproductive and only encourage the pseudo-myopia to intensify. We review concepts of visual hygiene and implement a vision therapy program. At the very least, the auto-refractor helps JL's parents understand the variable nature of JL's condition and helps account for some apparent inconsistencies in his performance.

Subjective

Case History, Including Signs, Symptoms, and Visual Needs
Cases of latent hyperopia can present with symptoms similar to those of pseudomyopia. Rather than distance blur, however, the presenting symptoms may be limited to visual discomfort. MC, a 12-year-old girl, initially was evaluated in our office 8 months ago. At that time, there were concerns about school performance, but MC had no visual symptoms. She previously had been given a spectacle lens prescription of OD +0.75 − 0.50 × 90 and OS +1.00 −0.50 × 90 but confessed that she rarely used the glasses because she was more comfortable without them and did not understand the need to wear them. Unaided visual acuity was 20/20 (6/6) at distance and near OD, OS, and OU. Manifest autorefractor find-ings at that time were as follows:

OD: +0.25 −0.00 × 0 (9)
    +0.50 −0.00 × 0 (9)
    +0.25 −0.25 × 10 (9)
OS: +1.00 −0.75 × 149 (9)
    +0.75 −0.75 × 151 (9)
    +1.00 −0.75 × 145 (9)

All binocular findings were normal, including tests of accommodative and vergence facility. The Keystone Visual Skills profile, conducted in our office as a standard portion of preliminary test data, was normal. At the present time, 8 months later, MC returns to our office with a chief complaint of headaches associated with near work. The Keystone Visual Skills profile now shows an eso shift at distance with normal phoria at near, arousing suspicion of latent hyperopia. Manifest refraction reveals the following findings:

OD: +0.25 –0.25 × 12 (9)
     –0.25 –0.50 × 151 (8)
     –0.50 –0.25 × 153 (8)
OS: +0.50 –0.50 × 139 (9)
     +0.50 –0.50 × 141 (9)
     +0.00 –0.50 × 133 (9)

The variability of the three findings in sphere, cylinder, and axis of the right eye and the lowered confidence value increase the suspicion of accommodative fluctuation secondary to latent hyperopia. Although we can infer this with near-point retinoscopy and other forms of near-point analysis, cycloplegic autorefraction readings pinpoint the latent hyperopia with greater precision. Before instilling cycloplegic drops, we trial frame +0.50 sphere OU to obtain MC's subjective impression, and she reports feeling more comfortable with the lenses at distance and particularly when looking at near print. Cycloplegic autorefraction with 1% cyclopentolate confirm bilateral latent hyperopia, as follows:

OD: +1.50 –0.25 × 180 (9)
     +1.25 –0.00 × 0 (9)
     +2.00 –0.50 × 132 (8)
OS: +1.75 –0.50 × 119 (9)
     +1.25 –0.50 × 159 (9)
     +1.25 –0.50 × 148 (9)

As noted in Chapter 5, when there is considerable variability in low amounts of cylinder, we prefer to prescribe a spherical lens correction. Although +0.50 sphere OU is close to the spherical equivalent prescription MC was given formerly, it proved to be a more effective prescription. We conduct a follow-up evaluation on MC 1 month later, and her headaches are reduced considerably. Manifest autorefraction is as follows:

OD: +0.25 –0.00 × 0 (9)
    +0.50 –0.25 × 10 (9)
    +0.50 –0.25 × 10 (9)
OS: +0.75 –0.50 × 158 (9)
    +0.75 –0.75 × 151 (9)
    +1.00 –0.50 × 161 (9)

These findings indicate a return toward the values recorded when MC originally was seen in our office. For many patients with latent hyperopia, the asymptomatic state is associated with manifest refraction in the range of low hyperopia, with internal consistency of repeated measures in each eye and high confidence values during autorefraction.

Subjective

Case History, Including Signs, Symptoms, and Visual Needs

We take a giant leap from the subtle changes in accommodation to the more dramatic interference in refraction that occurs with degradation of the crystalline lens due to cataract. IP, a 78-year-old retired optometrist, presented with a chief complaint of increasing glare at night while driving and a general sense that his acuity was decreasing. His wife is increasingly concerned about his hesitancy in identifying signs while driving. She accompanies him to the visit to make sure he tells us that his visual judgment at night is noticeably impaired.

His habitual lens prescription is

OD: –1.00 –2.00 × 90/+3.00
OS: Plano –3.00 × 90/+3.00

Through his prescription, his acuity is reduced to 20/50 (6/15) in the right eye and 20/40 +2 (6/12 +2) in the left eye. Manifest autorefraction is as follows:

OD: −0.25 −2.75 × 99 (7)
     −0.25 −2.75 × 98 (7)
     −0.25 −2.75 × 99 (6)
OS: +0.50 −3.25 × 85 (8)
     +0.50 −3.25 × 85 (8)
     +0.50 −3.25 × 85 (8)

There is no improvement in acuity on subjective refraction. The confidence values of the autorefraction readings match the biomicroscopic appearance, being lower in the right eye, where the cataract is denser. We therefore refer IP to a surgeon for cataract extraction and intraocular lens implantation. The operations on both eyes were conducted within 1 week of each other. Two weeks after the second eye was operated on, the manifest autorefraction is as follows:

OD: +0.75 −1.25 × 135 (8)
     +0.75 −1.25 × 137 (9)
     +0.75 −1.25 × 134 (8)
OS: −0.25 −0.75 × 166 (9)
     −0.25 −0.75 × 163 (9)
     Plano −0.75 × 171 (9)

Subjective refraction is

OD: +0.75 −1.25 × 135, providing 20/25 (6/7.5)
OS: −0.25 −0.75 × 165, providing 20/25 +2 (6/7.5 +2)

Automated refraction therefore can be used preoperatively to support the need for surgery due to image degradation based on reduced confidence values. It also can be used postoperatively to confirm distance power based in part on the repeatability of measures, as well as higher confidence values for each measure.

An IOL (intraocular lens) setting is incorporated into most auto-refractors to account for the presence of an intraocular implant.

Subjective

Case History, Including Signs, Symptoms, and Visual Needs
KB, the 51-year-old dean of a local university, presents to our office with a chief complaint of reduced visual acuity at distance and near. She reports seeing better if she rotates her head slightly sideways, looking through her glasses off-axis. Her eyes have been feeling "out of synch," and she is conscious of relying on the right eye more than the left. Lensometry showed her habitual prescription to be

OD: –3.00 –1.00 × 10/+2.25
OS: –3.00 –0.75 × 95/+2.25

Distance visual acuity through KB's habitual prescription is 20/20 –2 (6/6 –2) OD and 20/40 (6/12) OS. Manifest autorefraction is as follows:

OD: –2.75 –1.25 × 23 (8)
    –2.50 –1.50 × 19 (9)
    –2.75 –1.00 × 16 (9)
OS: –2.50 –2.50 × 125 (E)
    –2.00 –2.25 × 108 (7)
    –2.00 –2.75 × 109 (E)
    –1.50 –2.50 × 99 (7)
    –2.25 –2.25 × 108 (7)

Subjective refraction yields

OD: –2.75 –1.00 × 10/+2.25, providing 20/20 –1 (6/6 –1)
OS: –2.25 –2.25 × 105/+2.25, providing 20/25 (6/7.5)

Although we can identify various early phases of keratoconus with corneal topography and more advanced stages through distortion in keratometric mires, the autorefractor adds two important pieces of data. In the early phases, expect the confidence value to be reduced, and in the later phases to identify "error" measurements. More important, it provides a starting point for subjective refraction as compared to the scissors reflex obtained on manual retinoscopy.

In deciding to prescribe the full subjective refraction, we carefully consider two clinical pearls. **Clinical pearl 6** cautions against making asymmetrical prescription changes. Since KB presents with a strong feeling of the left eye being out of the picture and the right eye being fine, we feel secure in making a significant asymmetrical change in her habitual prescription. **Clinical pearl 8** advises that, "In making a lens change of more than 1 diopter, it often is prudent to prescribe the change in stages." Even though the spherical equivalent changes in KB's left lens was less than 1 diopter from the habitual prescription and even though in Chapter 5, on astigmatism, we caution against making large changes in cylinder power or axis, trial framing proves that KB is comfortable with the change.

KB returned for routine examination 1 year later, and although she still is pleased with her prescription from the previous year, manifest autorefraction now is

OD: –3.50 –1.25 × 5 (7)
$\quad$ –3.25 –1.50 × 9 (7)
$\quad$ –3.50 –1.50 × 10 (6)
OS: –1.25 –3.50 × 112 (8)
$\quad$ –1.25 –3.75 × 113 (7)
$\quad$ –1.25 –3.75 × 116 (5)

Subjective refraction yields

OD: –3.00 –1.00 × 9/+2.50, providing 20/25 –1 (6/7.5 –1)
OS: –1.75 –3.25 × 105/+2.50, providing 20/25 (6/7.5)

Based on the clinical examination, I advise KB that she is developing keratoconus in the right eye as well. She does not appreciate any substantial improvement through the subjective and decides not to change her prescription at this time.

KB returns 6 months later, stating that the right eye is worse than the left, and her best corrected spectacle lens acuity is 20/30 –3 (6/9 –3). The autorefractor keeps whirling during autoretinoscopy, unable to find an endpoint, recording multiple values of E.

Paradoxically, the left eye appears to have improved, showing the following:

OS: –3.25 –1.50 × 142 (7)
         –3.25 –1.75 × 126 (E)
         –3.00 –1.75 × 138 (8)
         –3.25 –1.25 × 132 (8)

Subjective refraction of the left eye now results in 20/25 +2 (6/7.5 +2) distance acuity, and we change KB's left spectacle lens accordingly. It is worth noting that **clinical pearl 17** suggests that, "The patient should understand the prognosis of his or her eye condition." In most cases of keratoconus, it is reasonable to advise the patient that the condition is expected to slowly worsen until a contact lens is necessary. In advanced cases, surgery may be indicated. Better to have a pleasant surprise, as with KB's left eye improving, than have the patient upset and concerned that acuity is worsening when unprepared for that likelihood.

Because the right eye no longer could be corrected satisfactorily with a spectacle lens, we refer her to a colleague who specializes in contact lenses, and KB is fit with a keratoconic lens for the right eye only. The contact lens restores acuity to 20/20 –2 (6/6 –2), and we prescribe a spectacle lens for the right eye of plano with a +2.50 add. To date, KB has remained comfortable and stable with this arrangement. The autorefractor proved to be a reliable index to fluctuations in refraction due to corneal changes and helped guide us to the best spectacle lens refraction and ultimately the need for contact lens correction.

Subjective

Case History, Including Signs, Symptoms, and Visual Needs
Periodically, the autorefractor yields spurious objective results. The most common source of error is overminusing patients with

active accommodation. In other instances, there is no apparent reason why the spherocylinder equivalent is significantly different from the subjective refraction. Experienced refractionists note that the same phenomenon occurs periodically with traditional retinoscopy. This apparently is the case with patient PW, a 53-year-old asymptomatic parking garage manager. He presents to the office for routine examination, having had his last eye examination 3 years ago. Lensometry showed his habitual prescription to be

OD: +1.25 –1.00 × 90 / +2.25
OS: +0.75 sphere / +2.25

Visual acuity through the habitual prescription is 20/20 (6/6) OD, OS, and OU at distance and near. Manifest autorefraction is as follows:

OD: +0.75 –1.00 × 87 (9)
      +1.00 –1.00 × 86 (9)
      +1.00 –1.25 × 88 (9)
OS: –0.25 –0.75 × 76 (9)
      –0.25 –1.00 × 105 (9)
      –0.25 –1.00 × 110 (9)

However, PW's subjective refraction proves to be the same as his habitual lens prescription. Therefore, be mindful of **clinical pearl 14**, "It is difficult to improve on the asymptomatic state." The autorefractor, with a high degree of confidence, indicates that PW would be happier with less plus sphere in both eyes and cylinder for the left eye. However, to avoid taking a risk in trying to convince PW that he is unhappy with his habitual lens prescription, we reissue his habitual lens prescription.

The Interface of Autophorometry and Autoretinoscopy

The autophorometer, at first blush appearing to add merely bells and whistles to the manual phoropter, provides distinct advantages.

It can be used independent of an autorefractor and autolensometer but the linkage of these three devices through a central interface is the prototypical design that makes commercially available integrated autorefraction systems so attractive.

In discussing the features that streamline autorefraction, we again limit ourselves to the Nidek system, with which we have the most clinical experience. However, the principles involved generalize to the other systems as well. An assistant neutralizes the patient's habitual prescription with the autolensometer (LM), after which autoretinoscopic findings are obtained through the autorefractor. Inside the instrument, a target simulates distance viewing, in this case a hot air balloon at the end of a highway. The examiner may elect to manually monitor the position of the eye when fixation is poor but more often can use the autoalignment feature. With a cooperative patient, readings of both eyes can be obtained within seconds. Difficulty collecting the data may be attributed to one of the variables listed in Table 2-1, in which case we ask the assistant to alert the doctor, but this is rare.

With the objective data collection phase completed and the patient seated behind the autophoropter, the examiner imports the data through a central control module. It is easiest to conceptualize this as the CPU (central processing unit) of the automated refraction system. The centerpiece CPU is visibly impressive from a practice management standpoint and has design features that enable the examiner to facilitate the refraction process. The touch of a single button or icon imports the patient's best-fit autoretinoscopic findings in sphere, cylinder, and axis from the autorefractor to the autophoropter in front of the right and left eyes simultaneously. It is most efficient, as well as most impressive, to have an automated projector linked with this arrangement. The projector we use is the Marco CP-670 and the initial presentation to the patient is the polarized slide that affords binocular refraction. This slide presents five letters decreasing in size from 20/50 to 20/20, so that an immediate impression can be gained in how close the autoretinoscopy comes to providing good visual acuity.

Although it is possible for the doctor to preprogram the flow of the refraction so that it is identical for each patient, we wish to emphasize the flexibility and power of the system. One can use the bichrome test for sphere and refine cylinder power and axis through either the traditional Jackson crossed-cylinder (JCC) test with a fan dial chart or a Simultans test. This allows the patient to select the preferred cylinder power and axis without having to respond to the familiar conundrum of "which is better, one or two." Our purpose here is not to discuss the Simultans test but to note that the simultaneity of refractive options to the patient is an important feature of the authophoropter.

When the subjective refraction has been determined, we enter this value into the CPU by pushing the "subjective" icon. The examiner then can import the patient's autolensometry finding in sphere, cylinder, and axis in front of both eyes simultaneously so that swift comparisons can be made:

Choice 1. Habitual lens prescription.
Choice 2. Autorefractor findings.
Choice 3. Subjective refraction.

When we import each of these choices through the CPU by selecting the appropriate icon, the sphere, cylinder, and axis are set in front of the right and left eyes simultaneously, within a second or two. The simultaneity of this change allows the patient to more validly compare the difference between the habitual prescription and the tentative prescription. If the patient favors the habitual lens prescription compared to the subjective, the tentative prescription can be changed and reentered into the CPU as the "final" prescription. The examiner then presents a choice between the habitual prescription and the "final" prescription. It may seem trivial to an examiner who has not had the opportunity to experience this process from the patient's side of the autophoropter, but the ability to make these instantaneous comparisons facilitates the patient's selection.

We summarize to the patient as follows:

Choice 1 (LM icon). This is the power that you have in your current glasses.
Choice 2 (AR icon). This is amount of power that the computer determined would make you see the sharpest when looking

at a distant target, and it is what we would prescribe if you were a robot.

Choice 3 (final icon). But, since you are not, you and I agreed on which lens prescription makes you feel most comfortable, which is this.

When the patient has no habitual prescription the examiner can enter the "unaided" icon, which allows the patient to choose between the unaided state and the final refraction value for direct comparison. When the patient wears contact lenses and we are conducting an overrefraction, the unaided icon is used to compare the contemplated change in power with the habitual state. In a paperless environment, the final prescription can be transferred to the patient's computer file and transcribed for laboratory processing with no possibility of manual transcription errors. As an aside, the autophoropter has another advantage in its centralized control of prism. With the control of one knob or icon, the examiner can increase or decrease the prism by equal amounts in front of both eyes simultaneously. This ensures that the prism vergence demand presented is both symmetrical and time regulated (smooth) as well as properly identified for base direction.

Delegation of Refraction

To address this topic, we first distinguish between objective and subjective refraction, then differentiate refraction from the art of prescribing lenses or prisms. After considering the material in this chapter, there should be little doubt that objective refraction can be delegated to a capable technician or assistant, in much the same way that automated visual fields can be delegated. The technology available allows the data to be collected with a high degree of confidence and reliability. The experienced examiner can look at the data and analyze its accuracy in the same way an examiner might sort out the realities from the artifacts of visual field data collected by an assistant. The principal difference lies in the interaction required between doctor and patient to determine the final prescription.

As gleaned from other chapters in this text and particularly from the pearls of conventional wisdom, the experienced practitioner often can predict what the final prescription will be based on the habitual lens prescription and the patient's case history. The job of the technician or assistant, particularly when using automated equipment, is to obtain the most accurate responses possible from the patient. With appropriate training, this might be done all the way to the point of determining the patient's final prescription. To do that, however, the doctor must call on a body of knowledge that goes beyond the training and experience of a technician. Indeed, this is a part of the professional judgment that differentiates the doctor from the technician.

For example, if the doctor senses or knows that the patient is sensitive to very small changes in lens power, the final prescription given may be very different from the values found on either objective or subjective refraction. For the foreseeable future, it will remain for the doctor to decide how much spherocylindrical change the patient tolerates best. Judgment about factors such as the impact of lens changes on accommodation or binocular vision, adaptation to change in habitual visual space including anticipated perceptual distortion with cylindrical changes, and the influence on ranges of clarity at near and intermediate distances can and should be made by the practitioner. Even when the decision is made that the prescription need not be changed, it is important for the doctor to explain how and why this is determined.

The art of prescribing lenses remains in the province of the practitioner, and listening to the patient's response to a contemplated change in prescription is as close as one gets to a "laying on of hands" in refraction. We suspect that some patients would be satisfied with final prescriptions derived from a set of standing orders executed through automated sequences. However, the time spent with the patient demonstrating and discussing proposed prescription changes helps maximize patient satisfaction and minimize the need for after-the-fact problem solving.

References

1. Milder B, Rubin ML. *The Fine Art of Prescribing Glasses without Making a Spectacle of Yourself.* Gainesville, FL: Triad Publishing Company, 1991:1.

2. Rosenberg R. Automated refraction. In: JB Eskridge, JF Amos, JD Bartlett (eds). *Clinical Procedures in Optometry.* Philadelphia: J.B. Lippincott 1991:168–173.
3. Grosvenor T. *Primary Care Optometry*, 4th ed. Boston: Butterworth–Heinemann, 2002:247.
4. Berman M, Nelson P, Caden B. Objective refraction: Comparison of retinoscopy and automated technique. *Am J Optom Physiol Opt.* 1994;61:204–209.
5. Sunder RP, Villada JR, Myint K, Lewis AE, Akingbehin T. Clinical evaluation of automated refraction in anterior chamber pseudophakia. *Br J Ophthalmol.* 1991;75:42–44.
6. Bennett AG, Rabbetts RB. *Clinical Visual Optics.* Boston: Butterworth–Heinemann, 1991:421–441.
7. Miwa T. Instrument myopia and the resting state of accommodation. *Optom Vis Sci.* 1992;69:55–59.
8. Borish IM, Catania LJ. Traditional versus computer-assisted refraction: Which is better? *J Am Optom Assoc.* 1997;68:749–756.
9. Gailmard NB, Sapposnek R. Should technicians refract? *Optom Management.* 1998:29-S–32-S.
10. West WD, Castells D. Which is better? Technicians performing automated-assisted refractions or optometrists performing phoropter-based refractions? *Rev Optometry.* 2001;138(3):82–86.
11. Marg E. *Computer-Assisted Eye Examination: Background and Prospects.* San Francisco: San Francisco Press, 1980:6.
12. Salvensen S, Kohler M. Automated refraction: Comparative study of automated refraction with the Nidek AR-1000 autorefractor and retinoscopy. *Acta Ophthalmol.* 1991;69:342–46.
13. Apell RJ. Clinical application of bell retinoscopy. *J Am Optom Assoc.* 1975;46:1023–1027.

CHAPTER 3

Prescribing for the Patient with Myopia

In Dickens-like fashion, Grosvenor and Goss preface their book on the clinical management of myopia by professing that myopia is both the easiest and one of the most difficult problems a vision care practitioner must treat.[1] Our clinical experience mirrors this observation. Myopia can be approached in either a very straightforward manner by simply prescribing the lens power providing sharp distance visual acuity or, in a more conservative and sophisticated manner, by taking into account patient comfort and the probabilities of contributing to myopic progression. As further noted by Grosvenor and Goss, anything a practitioner might be able to do to limit the development or progression of myopia is not simply lessening dependence on prescriptive lenses but helping to reduce the risk of the retinal detachment, chorioretinal degeneration, and glaucoma associated with myopic eyes.

More than with other refractive anomalies, our clinical model of the origin of myopia and myopic progression influences the nature of the prescription given to the patient.[2] One of the better synopses on this issue was provided by Rosner and Rosner,[3] and here we excerpt a few of their insightful observations:

> The argument over the control of the course of myopia through the manipulation of the lens prescription goes on. . . . There is clear need for continued scientific inquiry. The notion that the course of myopia is influenced at least to some degree by the amount of close work a patient engages in is not absurd. Many optometrists are convinced of a cause-

effect link between prolonged close work and myopia. The empirical evidence provided by their patients is too compelling to ignore, and the implications of the above-cited reports regarding dual innervation to the ciliary muscle, and differences in tonic accommodation between hyperopes, emmetropes, and early- and late-onset myopes seems to lend support to their speculations.

A detailed treatment of the functional view of myopia is well beyond the scope of this chapter, but we intermingle some functional or behavioral perspectives as they relate to specific case examples. During the past decade, a wealth of sources have organized and systematized thoughts about the impact of the environment on visual function in general and myopia in particular, and the reader is encouraged to peruse them.[4-8] To gain an appreciation for the unsolved issues regarding myopia control and its implications for prescribing lenses, consult the textbook edited by Rosenfield and Gilmartin.[9] Many aspects of myopia have attracted the interest of researchers from all over the world, as evidenced by the breadth of topics relating to the etiology and clinical correlates of myopia development and progression.[10] As with most clinical conditions, although the risk factors for myopia development cannot be given with absolute certainty, potential risk factors are widely agreed on (Table 3-1).

Table 3-1   Possible Risk Factors for Development of Myopia

Family history of myopia

Emmetropia before entry into school

Against-the-rule astigmatism

Abnormal accommodative function

Near-point esophoria

Chronic, sustained near work

Obstruction to image formation during infancy

Steep cornea or high axial length/cornea ratio

Source: Adapted from *Optometric Clinical Practice Guideline: Care of the Patient with Myopia*. St. Louis: American Optometric Association 1997:8.

Parents, particularly those with myopia, often are concerned about the likelihood of their children developing myopia. Are there any general trends we can cite with confidence? One of the better guides through which clinicians can counsel parents on their child's chances for developing myopia was provided by Zadnik and her colleagues.[11] Most children begin their school years with a low amount of hyperopia. As indicated in Figure 3-1, a child who still has at least 0.50 diopter of hyperopia in the third grade has a very low probability of developing myopia. The greater the amount of hyperopia at that age, the less likely the child is to progress into myopia. However, as soon as the child crosses the +0.50 threshold, the probability of progressing into myopia increases exponentially. For example, the child who is emmetropic in third grade has a 40% chance of developing myopia. Exhibiting as low as 0.25 diopter of myopia increases the probability that more myopia will develop to a 60% level. If 0.50 diopter of myopia is present at that age, the probability of developing at least 1 diopter of myopia increases to 80%.

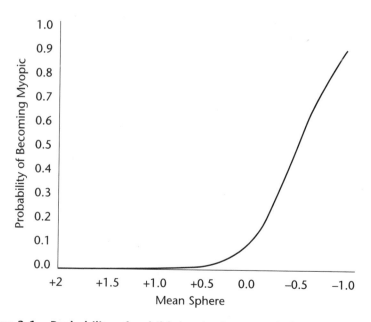

Figure 3-1 **Probability of a child developing myopia based on the refractive error in third grade.**

Clinical Guidelines in Prescribing for Myopia

Prescribing minus for sharpest distance clarity satisfies the majority of patients and reflects the maxim, "keep them in the green and they'll keep you in the green," as addressed in **clinical pearl 7**. This is the philosophy most of us learned in school, prescribing lenses for myopic patients that biases them slightly toward the green side of the chart when doing a bichrome balance. Throughout the years, researchers have suggested that this is the norm and any departure from full minus at distance would have to be defended. In this chapter, we consider prescriptive approaches to myopia other than full minus lens power at distance.

We begin by making the following bold statement and defending it, prior to discussing clinical tenets of prescribing for patients with myopia:

> The principles that constrain research on myopia control are the principles that make clinicians successful in prescribing for myopia. This is not meant to be offensive or curmudgeonly toward research, some of which can be very helpful in delineating population trends and guidelines. It is merely that, in clinical research trials, one must treat all the patients or subjects in a given treatment group the same. Patients typically are treated in a homogeneous manner once they are randomly assigned to a specific group, and the lens prescription given to the patient is derived arbitrarily.

As an example, look at how studies of the effectiveness of bifocals on the progression of myopia are conducted and how well they relate to clinical guidelines in prescribing bifocals for nonpresbyopic patients. A representative study recently published involves a randomized trial of the effect of single-vision versus bifocal lenses on myopia progression in children with esophoria.[12] The study was well conceived in limiting its population to children with esophoria, as previous studies have demonstrated that the rate of myopic progression slows more in patients with esophoria than exophoria.[13] However, an add of +1.50 was arbitrarily given to each child in the bifocal group. The rate of progression for each group then was analyzed and the authors concluded that the overall rate of progression in the bifocal group was modestly better than the single-vision group.

The problem with this approach is that a clinician deciding to prescribe a bifocal lens for a child would no sooner go with a "one size fits all" approach than arbitrarily select the same lens type or diameter for every contact lens patient. As elaborated elsewhere, multiple clinical tests that individualize a patient's near-point plus lens acceptance profile help predict in advance which children would benefit from an add.[14] Researchers could conduct the same type of evaluation that allows clinicians to derive an optimal near-point power and use that add rather than an arbitrary power[15] (Table 3-2). This would likely account for why some children seem to have their rate of myopia progression slowed by an add and others do not.[16] As noted by Wick, patients in myopia progression studies who are given an arbitrary add rather than an individualized add to reduce their lag of accommodation may simply adjust their near working distance and override the effect of the bifocal.[17]

A national consensus panel on care of the patient with myopia recommends that the correction of any significant degree of simple myopia that improves distance acuity be given to adolescents and adults (see Figure 3-1). However, the same consensus panel also recommends that parents of children with simple myopia be told about the options available for possible myopia control or reduction. For myopia induced by accommodative problems or other causes, the panel recommends that treatment be directed toward the cause of the myopia. This leads the practitioner to a closer look at the potential role of lenses in the containment of

Table 3-2   Data Sets of Plus Lens Acceptance at Near

NRA higher than PRA

Plus lens facility greater than minus lens facility

High lag of accommodation on near retinoscopy

Positive subjective response to added plus at near

N.P.C. or stereopsis improves with added plus lenses

Cycloplegia shows reduction in myopia >0.50 D

NRA, negative relative accommodation; PRA, positive relative accommodation.

myopia. We consider the role of RGP lenses as a modality in Chapter 8, on refractive care of the contact lens patient, and limit our focus in this chapter to the lens prescription itself.

With that background in mind, we offer the following general guidelines based on our combined clinical experiences. In a sense, they may be considered a myope's "Bill of Rights."

1. Most patients with myopia who have prescription lenses and complain of increased distance blur can be managed effectively by simply increasing the power in one or both eyes by a spherical equivalent power of –0.25 or –0.50.
2. Place the tentative increased prescription in a trial frame and have the patient confirm that objects or print at a distance not only look sharper but that the increase in power feels comfortable. Do not push an increase of 0.75 or higher when the patient would have been happy with less of an increase in power.
3. Listen to and respect your patient who tells you that he or she does not wish to have things "too sharp" at distance. Although many myopic patients want crystal clarity at distance, some are most comfortable with less minus than it takes to see a fly on the wall at a hundred yards.
4. Pre-presbyopic patients sometimes show a decrease in minus lens power at distance. However, **clinical pearl 5** cautions against reducing minus at distance with a myopic patient. Particularly when refracting in a relatively short room, we suggest trial framing the reduced power or, if it is a spherical reduction, simply holding plus trial lenses over the patient's current glasses and having him or her look out a window toward road or store signs to confirm that clarity is improved.
5. **Clinical pearl 14** advises that it is hard to improve upon an asymptomatic state. Patients given additional minus at distance simply because you measured it may find the lenses too strong, particularly for near work. If the patient is presbyopic, the unnecessary additional minus will reduce clarity at intermediate distances such as wall charts or the dashboard when driving.
6. Children in the early stages of myopia often can get by quite nicely without a lens prescription. Most children with my-

opia less than 1 diopter do not complain of distance blur. Such children can be managed by arranging a seat closer to the blackboard. However, once children complain of not being able to see the board effectively or even young children who exhibit more than 2 diopters of myopia, there is no virtue in withholding the prescription.

7. Undercorrect rather than fully correct a patient who exhibits accommodative or convergence excess. This may be a child with signs of functional myopia or pseudomyopia, particularly when demonstrating esophoria at near. The same holds true of any patient who does a considerable amount of sustained near work, as often occurs with computer use.

8. Be wary of pushing minus on a patient showing esophoria at distance with a high AC/A ratio. The additional lens power may result in double vision or increased eyestrain. Consider vision therapy or a low amount of base-out prism.

9. Some patients who experience increased myopia at night (large pupils with loss of depth of focus in darkness) may feel more secure in having a separate prescription for "glove compartment glasses." The prescription may have a spherical equivalent power of –0.25 or –0.50 diopter greater than their daytime distance glasses. The higher prescription may be of use also in poor weather during the daytime, when visibility otherwise would be compromised.

10. Deciding to prescribe an add for a nonpresbyopic patient rarely is based on subjective reports of near-point clarity but on a profile of near-point plus lens acceptance or to lessen esophoria. In general, a high lag of accommodation as determined with near retinoscopy or other lens findings will indicate plus lens acceptance. Data sets of plus lens acceptance are given in Table 3-2.

11. Prescribing a multifocal lens is more practical and effective than telling a student to remove her glasses when doing close work. Most children given a low or moderate minus lens prescription for distance will either wear the glasses or elect not to wear them. Most children advised to remove their glasses for near work simply forget to do so or find it a nuisance.

The Asymptomatic Myope

In guideline 6, we state that children in the early stages of myopia can often get by quite nicely without a lens prescription. Until driver's education, or more specifically when it's time to get behind the wheel, children with myopia less than 1 diopter rarely are faced with visual demands that would warrant a distance lens prescription. Consider patient JF, age 14, an outstanding student who has unaided acuity of 20/20 (6/6) with the right eye and 20/25+ (6/7.5+) in the left eye. He has the following retinoscopic findings:

OD: Plano −0.25 × 155
OS: −0.50 sphere

JF's subjective findings are plano in the right eye, and −0.25 sphere in the left eye to obtain 20/20 (6/6). If we were to consider preventive care to limit the development of myopia, the near-point findings would be of interest. The majority of eye care practitioners would not prescribe lenses nor see the relevance in gathering near-point data in a case like this other than to document fusion and perhaps accommodative amplitude. Birnbaum makes a strong argument for considering the gathering and application of near-point data to determine a possible near-point lens prescription for patients such as JF.[18]

Consider another child, this one younger and with a little more myopia. Patient GF is a 9-year-old child whose mother brings him in for routine examination. He is a good student with no developmental abnormalities, and his distance clarity seems fine. However, his mother is concerned because both she and the boy's father began wearing glasses at age 9. She wants to know whether or not he is nearsighted yet. GF's unaided distance acuity is 20/30 (6/9) in each eye and 20/25 (6/7.5) with both eyes together. His retinoscopic findings are as follows:

OD: −1.00 −0.25 × 90
OS: −1.00 −0.75 × 105

Keratometric readings are spherical in the right eye and 0.50 against-the-rule astigmatism in the left eye. GF's subjective refraction is –0.50 sph OU to obtain 20/20 (6/6) in each eye. Again, we could make the case for considering plus lens application at near if the near-point findings warrant it, particularly if the child shows esophoria at near.[19] Our experience has been that the majority of eye care practitioners would counsel his mother that GF is going to become progressively more nearsighted independent of attempts to slow myopic progression. Once myopia appears in childhood, it inevitably increases in amount.[20]

Our clinical experience has been that, in general, it is reasonable to conclude that children of highly myopic parents are destined to become myopic given the genetic predisposition and the influence of near work. When neither parent is appreciably myopic, it is more reasonable to be aggressive about myopia control. When one parent is appreciably nearsighted, all bets are off. Research into patterns of myopia onset and progression are ongoing and ultimately may provide guidelines that are more definitive than clinical impressions.

When leaving a myopic child who has failed a school vision screening uncorrected or undercorrected, it is important to let the school nurse know why you are choosing not to correct the child's acuity to 20/20 (6/6). Although there is ample reason to choose not to provide the sharpest distance acuity possible, most parents and school nurses will not expect or understand your reasoning unless you make note of it.[21]

Clinical pearl 14 as well as the fifth clinical guideline caution against attempts to improve on the asymptomatic state, particularly when an adult patient is wearing a lens prescription happily. Nevertheless, there are tempting options to consider in cases such as patient ME.

Subjective

Case History, Including Signs, Symptoms, and Visual Needs
ME is a 39-year-old postal worker, who takes birth control pills but no other medication, and her general health is excellent. The main purpose of her visit is for a routine eye examination and to obtain prescription sunglasses. ME mentions that her mother has glaucoma and that sister was recently told that she is suspect for

glaucoma. She is perfectly happy with her current glasses, which she wears full time. She has never worn, nor has any interest in wearing, contact lenses and is not interested in refractive surgery.

Lensometry
OD: −0.75 −1.50 × 10
OS: −2.00 −1.25 × 170

Objective

Ocular Health Assessment
Internal and external eye structures are healthy and normal in appearance, including C/D of 0.3/0.3 and good neuroretinal rims. Automated visual field screening and intraocular pressures are normal and angles are wide by Van Herrick estimation.

Clinical Measures

	At 20 ft (6 m)	At 16 in. (40 cm)
VA (cc):	OD: 20/25− (6/7.5−)	20/20 (6/6)
	OS: 20/20 (6/6)	20/25+ (6/7.5+)
Cover Test:	Ortho	Ortho
N.P.C.:	To nose	
Retinoscopy/	OD: −1.50 −1.75 × 11	
Autorefractor:	OS: −2.25 −1.50 × 173	
Subjective:	OD: −1.25 −1.75 × 10	VA 20/20 (6/6)
	OS: −2.00 −1.25 × 173	VA 20/20 (6/6)
Phoria:	Ortho	2 Exop
Base-in vergences:	N/E	N/E
Base-out vergences:	N/E	N/E
Accom. Amplitude:	6.50	
Neg. Rel. Accom.:	+2.00	
Pos. Rel. Accom.:	−1.50	
Fused X-Cyl.:	+0.50	
Stereo:	N/E	

Assessment

ME has compound myopic astigmatism with an anisometropic amount greater in the left eye.

Plan

1. We decided not to change ME's prescription. We wrote a prescription for her sunglasses that is identical to ME's habitual prescription.
2. We considered increasing the minus lens prescription of the right eye. An argument in favor of that approach would be that ME is going to be using the sunglasses primarily for distance and therefore should have the benefit of improved distance clarity in the right eye. There is a good chance that ME will have adaptive difficulty since she is happy with her current prescription. This is particularly true because she will be wearing her habitual prescription the majority of the time and readjusting to the higher minus in the right eye every time she puts her sunglasses on.
3. We could suggest that ME change her prescription to increase the minus lens value of the right eye for both her regular glasses and sunglasses, but again we asked ourselves, "Why try to convince ME that she's not happy with her current prescription?"

Conventional Myopia

The conventional myope is one who presents with a chief complaint of distance blur that does not vary. There is no fluctuation in distance vision after extended periods of close work, and there is no problem with blur at near. In virtually all these cases, the patient's chief concern can be addressed by simply increasing the spherical equivalent minus lens power in one or both lenses. Patient MG represents the conventional myope, the subgroup that constitutes the majority of myopic patients seen in practice.

Subjective

Case History, Including Signs, Symptoms, and Visual Needs
MG is a 24-year-old employee of a trucking company. He started with the company by helping to load trucks and now is on the road quite a bit. MG has designs on working his way up the ladder to management. His chief complaint is that road signs at

night, or even during the daytime when in unfamiliar areas, are not as sharp as they had been. You check his record and note that he was last examined in your office 2 years ago. He had the same complaint at that time and you increased his prescription by 0.25 diopter in each eye. Looking back further, you note that you gave him his first prescription in your office 12 years ago, and it was −0.50 sph OU.

Lensometry
OD: −1.50 sphere
OS: −1.25 sphere

Objective

Ocular Health Assessment
Internal and external eye structures were healthy and normal in appearance.

Clinical Measures

	At 20 ft (6 m)	At 16 in. (40 cm)
VA (cc):	OD: 20/25+ (6/7.5+)	20/20 (6/6)
	OS: 20/25+ (6/7.5+)	20/20 (6/6)
Cover Test:	Ortho	Ortho
N.P.C.:	To the nose	
Retinoscopy/	OD: −1.75 −0.25 × 135	
Autorefractor:	OS: −1.50 −0.25 × 130	
Subjective:	OD: −1.75 sphere	VA 20/20
	OS: −1.50 sphere	VA 20/20
Phoria:	Ortho	2 Esop
Base-in vergences:	N/E	X/18/14
Base-out vergences:	N/E	N/E
Accom. Amplitude:	9.00	
Neg. Rel. Accom.:	+2.25	
Pos. Rel. Accom.:	−2.50	
Fused X-Cyl.:	+0.50	
Stereo:	N/E	

Assessment

MG has simple myopia with mild and stable esophoria at near and a slow rate of myopic progression.

Plan

1. Prescribe new lenses, increasing the power in each eye by –0.25 sphere.
2. Neither you nor MG is concerned about the rate of progression of 0.25 in 2 years. Although he has esophoria at near, it has been present for 12 years and is not increasing, nor is he symptomatic at near. His compensatory (base in) vergence range at near is normal. He will return in 1–2 years for routine comprehensive eye examination, and from the very slow drift through the years, you can tell him to expect that future changes will be minimal.

Near-Work-Induced Myopia

Clinicians have long recognized that sustained periods of near work tends to induce myopia in susceptible individuals and that the prescribing of minus lenses may contribute to the progression of myopia.[22] Applied research suggests that accommodation plays a critical role in the progression of myopia.[23–25] Ciuffreda and Ordonez established that abnormal transient myopia in symptomatic individuals occurs after sustained near work and transient distance blur after near work decreases progressively and markedly through optometric vision therapy that improves accommodative facility.[26] In the absence of such therapy, the manner in which accommodation is influenced by lens prescription may play a key role in adaptive myopia, the progression of myopia, and its interrelationship with distance blur.[27,28]

In prescribing for near-work-induced myopia, it would be helpful to be able to identify which patients are most susceptible to adaptive myopiagenic influences. Also important to note is that an individual may have multiple types of myopia coexisting.[29] In other words, one can experience structural myopia, for which there is a genetic predisposition, and later experience functional or

Table 3-3   Suggestions for Visual Hygiene

Reading and writing activities at the Harmon distance*
Reading and writing on slant board at a 20° angle
Nonglare source of lighting and good posture
Computer screen viewing at 16–30 in. (40–75 cm)
Computer screen viewing angle 10–20° downward
15 minute break for each hour of computer use
20/20 rule: Shift to distance fixation for ≥20 seconds every 20 minutes

*Distance from mid-knuckle to elbow, estimated by placing an elbow on the table surface and resting the chin in the palm of that hand.

adaptive myopia due to prolonged near-point stress. Prescribing for the adaptive component of the myopia presents the opportunity to modify the overall prescription based on the patient's findings and behavioral response to spherical-, cylindrical-, or prismatic-lens-induced changes.[30] Suggestions for visual hygiene and other nonoptical forms of vision therapy complement alternative approaches to lens prescribing (Table 3-3).

Gathering visual data, including accommodation, phoria, and vergence findings and the study of their interrelationships, may help identify the patients experiencing near-work-induced or adaptive visual problems. Various systems of analysis are available, including OEP (Optometric Extension Program) analysis, graphical analysis including fixation disparity,[31] and integrative analysis.[32] Most clinicians decide on a particular form of analysis or other insights to determine the extent to which a patient's myopia is adaptive and, therefore, what lenses will be prescribed.

Phases of Progressive Myopia

If we accept the premise that some component of permanent myopia may have begun as transient myopia induced by near-point stress, is there a transitional phase where we might be more conservative in prescribing minus lenses for distance and more aggressive in prescribing plus lenses for near? Ong and Ciuffreda suggest that this might be the case.[33] Our clinical experience agrees with the theory that some cases of progressive myopia initially exhibit signs that are adaptive in nature and that a transitional phase occurs, during which transient pseudomyopia converts to permanent myopia.

For example, a patient who is old enough to offer a reliable history may tell you that when he or she first started to experience distance blur it was more noticeable following periods of sustained close work. However, after receiving the first minus lens prescription for distance and progressing toward more distance blur within a period of months, less fluctuation was noted and the blur at distance became constant. This observation is not new, having been introduced in OEP literature through the concept of embeddedness. Current research appears to validate the way functional practitioners have treated myopia for over 50 years (Table 3-4). Manas[34] elaborates four specific phases of acquired myopia, considered to be cyclic steps of adaptation:

1. *Daily recurrent vocational myopia.* This is equivalent to NITM (near-work-induced transient myopia). Clinical data show plus lens acceptance at near, and the prescription of plus lenses at near is likely to reverse the development of myopia.
2. *Fixed myopia with loss of distance acuity but still showing plus lens acceptance at near.* Minimum minus at distance to meet acuity requirements is recommended as well as whatever plus at near is acceptable.
3. *Increased myopia at distance with loss of plus lens acceptance at near.* Vision therapy would be necessary before the patient can accept an add, even if esophoria is exhibited. The prescription of

Table 3-4   Prescription Options for Myopia

Full distance prescription only
Full distance prescription with bifocal
Underprescribe for distance
Underprescribe for distance with bifocal
No distance prescription; plus lens for near

minus spheres alone usually speeds up progression through the myopic cycle.

4. *Stabilized myopic adaptation and use of the same minus lens prescription at distance and near with efficiency and comfort.* If increased efficiency at near is needed (new job with more near-point work or stress), the four-phase cycle may repeat itself.

Applications of Autorefraction and Cycloplegia

We use 1% cyclopentolate solution for routine cycloplegia when investigating pseudomyopia. Our emphasis here is on myopia due to accommodative excess rather than pseudomyopia in connection with night or empty field myopia. Accommodative excess may be mild, as in near-work-induced transient myopia, or more severe, as occurs with intense accommodative spasm. There are numerous indicators of pseudomyopia (Table 3-5), the most obvious being that the patient experiences variable degrees of distance blur. Although the distance blur usually is exacerbated by periods of extended close work, it may occur spontaneously. The hallmark of pseudomyopia secondary to accommodative excess is the rapid reduction in myopia under cycloplegia. Most cases can be man-

Table 3-5   Clinical Indications of Pseudomyopia

Fluctuating distance vision
Distance vision blurrier after near work
Near acuity may be reduced but less than distance
Asthenopia or brow ache if intense spasm
Pupillary fluctuation or constriction if intense spasm
Often accompanied by clinical history of anxiety
Minus lenses do not provide as much clarity as expected
Flashes of higher myopia on retinoscopy/autorefraction
Intermittent esophoria or esotropia if high AC/A
Constricted NRA/PRA and accommodative facility
Cycloplegic refraction shows considerably less myopia

NRA, negative relative accommodation; PRA, positive relative accommodation.

aged effectively with a plus lens prescription for near, sometimes in conjunction with active vision therapy. In severe cases, we can relax accommodation with cycloplegia therapeutically.[35]

Mental state, particularly anxiety or anger, can result in involuntary accommodative excess.[36] The comparison of manifest and cycloplegic findings, particularly when documented with a printout of autorefractor findings, makes it easier for the examiner to explain the findings to the patient. Chapter 2 provides specific examples of this. Some clinicians suggest that it is foolish to use cycloplegia, even as an adjunct to refraction.[37] As we demonstrate, in most cases of pseudomyopia, it is foolish not to do a cycloplegic refraction. We now look at several cases of pseudomyopia where the diagnosis and management was guided by the results of autorefraction in conjunction with cycloplegia. Our approach in these cases is to treat near-point findings as supplemental. In most instances, the patient history and refractive findings are sufficient to make the diagnosis. We begin with patient CG.

Subjective

Case History, Including Signs, Symptoms, and Visual Needs

CG is a 12-year-old child who is an excellent student and a budding cello player. Her habitual working distance is at 24 in. (60 cm). For the past few months, CG has noticed that, after reading for awhile, whether schoolwork or music notes, objects across the room are blurrier. When it first began, CG would notice the blur only after prolonged periods of close work and the distance blur cleared quickly. She is concerned now because the blur happens after a shorter period of time and persists longer.

Objective

Clinical Measures

	At 20 ft (6 m)	*At 16 in. (40 cm)*
VA (cc):	OD: 20/20 (6/6)	20/20 (6/6)
	OS: 20/20 (6/6)	20/20 (6/6)
Cover Test:	Ortho	Sl esop
N.P.C.:	1 in./3 in. (2.5 cm/7.5 cm) OS out; no diplopia	

Retinoscopy/	Manifest autorefraction,*
Autorefractor:	OD: 0.25 –0.50 × 104 (9)
	–0.75 –0.50 × 132 (9)
	–1.75 –0.25 × 134 (9)
	OS: –1.00 –0.50 × 122 (9)
	–0.50 –1.00 × 118 (9)
	–0.50 –0.75 × 124 (9)
	Cycloplegic autorefraction,
	OD: +0.75 –0.50 × 138 (9)
	+0.75 –0.50 × 141 (9)
	+0.50 –0.25 × 140 (9)
	OS: +0.75 –0.50 × 134 (9)
	+0.75 –0.50 × 133 (9)
	+0.50 –0.50 × 136 (9)

Subjective:	OD: Plano	VA 20/20 (6/6)
	OS : Plano	VA 20/20 (6/6)
	Additional near-point testing is N/E	

Assessment

Pseudomyopia with fluctuating distance acuity secondary to accommodative excess.

Plan

1. We decide to give CG a single vision prescription of +0.50 sphere OU for use primarily when reading or playing cello. She returns 1 month later, and we obtain the following findings for manifest autorefraction:

   OD: Plano –0.50 × 24 (9)
         –0.25 –0.25 × 172 (9)
         –0.50 –0.25 × 164 (9)
   OS: –0.50 –0.25 × 157 (9)
         –0.25 –0.50 × 145 (9)
         +0.25 –0.50 × 157 (9)

2. CG is happy about her ability to sustain accuracy in refocusing from near to distance for longer periods of time. We ask her to continue using the prescription lenses for all sus-

---

*Chapter 2 explains the function of confidence values as used with autorefraction.

tained visual tasks. CG has a low amount of latent hyperopia and responds readily to lenses alone.

Our next case, PR, is a bit more complex.

Subjective

Case History, Including Signs, Symptoms, and Visual Needs
PR is a 10-year-old child whose mother observed her to fatigue
quickly when reading. PR's reading tutor noticed the same thing;
and the mother's cousin, who benefited from vision therapy,
urged her to come to us for evaluation. PR previously had been
examined by two eye doctors, who prescribed glasses for astigmatism. We neutralized her glasses, neither of which she used, as
follows. First prescription,

OD: Plano –0.25 × 80
OS: Plano –0.25 × 170

Second prescription,

OD: Plano –0.25 × 80
OS: Plano –0.25 × 90

Objective

Clinical Measures

	At 20 ft (6 m)	*At 16 in. (40 cm)*
VA (cc):	OD: 20/20 (6/6)	20/20 (6/6)
	OS: 20/20 (6/6)	20/20 (6/6)
Cover Test:	Ortho	Sl esop
N.P.C.:	2 in./4 in. (5 cm/10 cm) OS out;	
	no diplopia	
Retinoscopy/	Manifest autorefraction,	
Autorefractor:	OD: +0.25 –0.75 × 74 (8)	
	–0.75 –0.75 × 61 (5)	
	–0.25 –0.75 × 79 (9)	
	OS: –2.75 –2.00 × 112 (5)	
	–2.75 –0.75 × 110 (9)	
	–1.50 –0.50 × 113 (9)	

Retinoscopy/	Cycloplegic autorefraction,
Autorefractor	OD: +1.25 –0.50 × 83 (9)
continued:	+1.25 –0.50 × 86 (9)
	+1.25 –0.50 × 83 (9)
	OS: +1.25 –0.75 × 103 (9)
	+1.00 –0.50 × 119 (9)
	+1.00 –0.50 × 120 (9)
Subjective:	OD: Plano VA 20/20 (6/6)
	OS: Plano VA 20/20 (6/6)
	Additional near-point testing is N/E

Assessment

Isometropic latent hyperopia with anisometropic accommodative spasm.

Plan

1. The assessment warrants a few words of explanation as a prelude to the plan. When looking at the manifest refraction, it is easy to note from some of the low confidence values, as well as PR's relatively high unaided acuity, that she experiences accommodative excess. Further, the amount of spasm appears to be significantly higher in the left eye than the right eye, based on the amount of minus. However, cycloplegic refraction shows that, in the relaxed state, PR actually is isometropic.

2. We decided that giving PR a lens prescription would be a shot in the dark. The reason we cite the case here is that sometimes the best decision you make about which lens to prescribe is no lens at all. While some children will be assuaged and some underlying problems resolved by the belief that a low astigmatic lens power will help, objective cycloplegic data can remove a lot of the guesswork.

3. We administered accommodative therapy, to which PR responded well. At the very least, the cycloplegic findings document that the patient and her parents should be counseled about the nature of accommodative excess and given suggestions for visual hygiene to minimize the symptoms.[38]

For some patients, accommodative excess is more than a nuisance imposed by variable blur. Pseudomyopia can impair an individual's lifestyle, as was the case with patient CC.

Subjective

Case History, Including Signs, Symptoms, and Visual Needs

CC is an 18-year-old local high school basketball star, who has a scholarship to play college ball. He is due to begin his freshman year in the fall but has significant difficulty in focusing clearly at any distance. He was evaluated by an optometric colleague working in a large ophthalmologic practice that specializes in refractive surgery. It is the end of June, and CC is at risk for losing his scholarship if he cannot focus accurately. CC has a long-standing history of color deficiency, but his eye examinations otherwise always had been normal until this year.

Lensometry
OD: $+0.50 -0.75 \times 80$
OS: $+0.50 -0.50 \times 75$

Objective

Ocular Health Assessment

Internal and external eye structures are healthy and normal in appearance.

Clinical Measures

		At 20 ft (6 m)	At 16 in. (40 cm)
VA (cc):	OD:	20/25 (6/7.5)	20/25 (6/7.5)
	OS:	20/30 (6/9)	20/30 (6/9)
Cover Test:		Sl esop	Sl esop
N.P.C.:		To the nose	
Retinoscopy/	OD:	$-4.25 -0.50 \times 77$ (9)	
Autorefractor		$-4.50 -0.50 \times 77$ (9)	
(manifest/dry):		$-4.75 -0.50 \times 98$ (9)	
	OS:	$-7.50 -0.25 \times 26$ (9)	
		$-7.50 -0.50 \times 174$ (9)	
		$-7.50 -0.25 \times 158$ (9)	

	At 20 ft (6 m)	*At 16 in. (40 cm)*
Subjective	OD: Plano	VA 20/25 (6/7.5)
(manifest/dry):	OS: Plano	VA 20/30 (6/9)
Retinoscopy/	OD: −0.75 −0.25 × 83 (9)	
Autorefractor	−1.50 −0.25 × 58 (9)	
(wet/cycloplegic):	−1.75 −0.25 × 71 (9)	
	OS: −1.75 sphere (9)	
	−1.00 −0.25 × 133 (9)	
	−2.00 −0.25 × 66 (9)	
Subjective	OD: Plano	VA 20/20 (6/6)
(wet/cycloplegic):	OS: Plano	VA 20/20 (6/6)
Phoria:	1 eso	2 eso
Base-in vergences	N/E	N/E
Base-out vergences	N/E	N/E
Accom. Amplitude:	N/E	
Neg. Rel. Accom.:	N/E	
Pos. Rel. Accom.:	N/E	
Fused X-Cyl.:	N/E	
Stereo:	N/E	

Assessment

CC has intense asymmetric accommodative spasm, alleviated by cycloplegia.

Plan

1. CC was not using the glasses initially prescribed because he did not perceive any benefit when wearing them.
2. Although we could have prescribed an add, even under cycloplegia CC shows a significant myopic shift. Given the short time frame in which the referring optometrist asks us to help, we decide to implement an intensive vision therapy program to get CC to the point where he can use a plus lens prescription at near to help keep his accommodative response in check.
3. Note that we omitted virtually all the near-point findings as unessential. The reason for doing so is that, with the manifest refraction showing significant accommodative excess and unaided acuities relatively clear, the diagnosis and

management direction are very clear. Our focus is on the cycloplegic findings to get an indication as to how readily CC would give up or relax the accommodative spasm. That helped us not only explain the condition to CC, his parents, and his coaches but establish a realistic time frame for therapy. We decided to change CC's prescription to +0.50 sph OU and asked him to use the lenses whenever he felt more comfortable, relaxed, or in better focus when putting them on.

4. CC began a vision therapy program in the beginning of July, during which he came to the office for 1 hour daily. We assign home activities to be done over the weekend, concentrating on a lot of accommodative flexibility therapy. CC rarely uses the near prescription. As the stability of his focusing rapidly improves, he simply forgets to put them on. He plays basketball daily with improved confidence. By the end of July, he had stable unaided acuity of 20/20 with either eye and manifest autorefractor findings as follows:
   OD: Plano –0.75 × 63 (8)
       Plano –0.50 × 91 (9)
       Plano –0.50 × 85 (9)
   OS: Plano –0.25 × 152 (9)
       Plano –0.25 × 168 (9)

5. CCs' final progress evaluation is on August 20. Unaided acuities are 20/20 with each eye, and manifest autorefractor findings are as follows:
   OD: Plano –0.25 × 58 (9)
       Plano –0.25 × 60 (9)
       Plano –0.25 × 72 (9)
   OS: Plano (9)
       Plano (9)
       Plano (9)

CC was never as happy to obtain so many "zeroes" on a test. We take near-point findings so that they can be used for reference in the future if CC feels like he is regressing, and we encourage him to use the +0.50 sph OU for all sustained visual activities. His near-point findings are as follows.

	At 20 ft (6 m)	*At 16 in. (40 cm)*
Phoria:	Ortho	1 eso
Base-in vergences:	X/10/4	X/18/14
Base-out vergences:	X/20/14	X/18/12
Accom. Amplitude:	10.00	
Neg. Rel. Accom.:	+2.25	
Pos. Rel. Accom.:	–2.50	
Fused X-Cyl.:	+0.75	
Stereo:	20 seconds of arc	

We have tracked CC since dismissing him to the care of his primary optometrist, and he remains symptom-free. His latest refraction is plano –0.75 × 60, but he feels no need for prescription lenses at distance or near. We emphasize that, although CC's case certainly could have been managed without an autorefractor or cycloplegia, utilizing both these tools gave us streamlined, objective data simplifying management of the case.

Although we would expect large amounts of pseudomyopia to be confined to children or adolescents, we have encountered patients with accommodative excess in their late thirties or forties, of whom NK is a striking example.

Subjective

Case History, Including Signs, Symptoms, and Visual Needs
NK is a 38-year-old woman who assists her husband with his home-based business.

She has a prior history of a C4–C5 herniated disc from a childhood injury and has been taking iron supplements for the past 14 years. When NK first consulted with us, she had been having severe bouts of dizziness, headaches, and pain in and around the eyes for 3 years. Neuroimaging studies were negative and treatment with medication such as Antivert was of no benefit. She had been evaluated and treated at an "eighth-nerve center" of a local hospital, including receiving vestibular therapy through the physical therapy department, all to no avail. NK also has a sensation that she is constantly fighting off the feeling of the right eye pulling inward. She had been given glasses by her previous eye doctor but felt worse with them than without them.

Lensometry

OD: +0.50 –0.25 × 90

OS: +0.50 sphere

Objective

Ocular Health Assessment

Internal and external eye structures are healthy and normal in appearance.

Clinical Measures

		At 20 ft (6 m)	*At 16 in. (40 cm)*
VA (cc):	OD:	20/20 (6/6)	20/20 (6/6)
	OS:	20/20 (6/6)	20/20 (6/6)
Cover Test:		Sl esop	Sl esop
N.P.C.:		To the nose	
Retinoscopy/		Manifest autorefraction,	
Autorefractor:	OD:	–1.25 –0.25 × 120 (9)	
		–1.75 sphere (9)	
		–1.75 –0.25 × 115 (9)	
	OS:	Plano –0.75 × 19 (9)	
		–0.50 –0.50 × 22 (9)	
		–0.50 –0.50 × 22 (9)	
		Cycloplegic autorefraction,	
	OD:	+2.75 –0.50 × 117 (9)	
		+2.75 –0.25 × 116 (9)	
		+2.75 –0.50 × 117 (9)	
	OS:	+3.00 –0.75 × 8 (9)	
		+3.00 –0.75 × 10 (9)	
		+3.00 –0.75 × 7 (9)	
Subjective (manifest):	OD:	Plano	VA 20/20
	OS:	Plano	VA 20/20
Phoria:		2 eso	3 eso
Base-in vergences:		N/E	X/4/2
Base-out vergences:		N/E	X/6/3

Note: Given the nature of NK's symptoms, we also measured the vertical phoria, which was ortho, and the supra- and infravergences, which were 2/1 in both directions.

Accom. Amplitude:	6.00
Neg. Rel. Accom.:	+0.50
Pos. Rel. Accom.:	–0.75
Fused X-Cyl.:	+0.50
Stereo:	40 seconds of arc

Assessment

NK has latent hyperopia with intense asymmetric accommodative spasm resulting in anisometropic pseudomyopia.

Plan

1. NK has constricted ranges in accommodation, lateral vergence, and vertical vergence.
2. We treat NK by encouraging her to wear her habitual prescription glasses full time rather than putting them on briefly and giving up. We also prescribe vision therapy to break the pseudomyopia and expand fusional vergence ranges.
3. We are successful in getting NK to wear a contact lens prescription of +0.50 sphere OU full time by fitting her with contact lenses. Through vision therapy, she is able to significantly expand accommodative and fusional vergence ranges in all directions. Manifest autorefractor findings stabilize at +0.50 sphere OD and +0.75 sphere OS. She feels wonderful for a period of 1 month; however, all NK's symptoms remain.

Even though objectively NK improves considerably, her subjective symptoms of dizziness and general visual sensitivity seem disproportionate to the amount of residual latent hyperopia. We conduct threshold visual fields, which are unremarkable, and refer NK to an optometric colleague for electroretinography (ERG) and visually evoked potential (VEP), both of which prove negative. Although we are successful in reducing NK's pseudomyopia, she still has residual accommodative excess to compensate for the full amount of latent hyperopia.

NK's case is striking for the amount of accommodative spasm that can be exhibited on the doorstep of presbyopia. In the next section, we consider the refractive implications of myopic shifts actually associated with early presbyopia.

Myopic Changes in Early Presbyopia

In early presbyopia, myopia can either increase, decrease, or remain stable. Shifts in myopia can occur in one or both eyes and may even increase in one eye and decrease in the fellow eye. Although stability in distance refraction is more common than fluctuation or change, the distance shifts in myopia provide the greater refractive challenges. Although rare, clinicians should be vigilant to myopic shifts associated with changes in the refractive index of the crystalline lens induced by pharmacological or systemic causes (Table 3-6). An increase in myopia can occur secondary to medications, most notably sulfonamides, diuretics, and

Table 3-6   Systemic Drugs Prone to Cause Transient Myopia

Acetazolamide
Hydrochlorothiazide
Tetracyclines
Prochlorperazine
Corticosteroids
Ampicillin
Acetaminophen
Arsenicals
Sulfonamides
Hydralazine
Ethoxzolamide
Oral contraceptives
Nonsteroidal anti-inflammatory drugs

Source: Adapted from Blaho KE, Connor CG, Winbery SL. Pharmacology and refraction. In: Benjamin WJ (ed). *Borish's Clinical Refraction*. Philadelphia: Saunders, 1998:384.

carbonic anhydrase inhibitors.[39] The transient increase in myopia associated with elevated blood glucose levels in diabetes has long been recognized, but a more recent consideration is the potential decrease in acuity associated with lens or pupillary damage unintentionally caused by panretinal laser surgery.[40]

As accommodative amplitude progressively lessens, the clinician occasionally encounters patients in early presbyopia who exhibit a pseudomyopic shift. Through efforts to maximize the accommodative response, some pre-presbyopic patients actually refract more minus at distance than before.[41] An example of this pseudomyopic shift in early presbyopia is presented in Chapter 5, in the case of a 43-year-old dentist, LL. There is also a flip side to this coin, however. What happens to patients who acquired pseudomyopia in adolescence or college years, which became embedded or locked in when minus lenses were prescribed to improve distance clarity? If the theory about functional myopia stemming from accommodative excess is correct, some portion of the accommodative excess should lessen with the reduction in accommodative response during the presbyopic years. This would result in the patient exhibiting less myopia and therefore experiencing near-point blur compounded by looking through a distance prescription that now contains more minus lens power than needed. This appears to be the case with patient JW.

Subjective

Case History, Including Signs, Symptoms, and Visual Needs
JW, a 44-year-old attorney, until recently wore glasses all the time. He does a great deal of reading and has developed the habit of removing his glasses when reading. His prior eye doctor told him last year that he was able to reduce the strength of the prescription to avoid the need for bifocals. JW's general health is excellent, and he takes no medications.

Lensometry
OD: $-1.75 -1.75 \times 20$
OS: $-2.75 -2.00 \times 180$

Objective

Ocular Health Assessment

Internal and external eye structures are healthy and normal in appearance.

Clinical Measures

		At 20 ft (6 m)	*At 16 in. (40 cm)*
VA (cc):	OD:	20/25+ (6/7.5+)	20/25 (6/7.5)
	OS:	20/25– (6/7.5–)	20/30 (6/9)
Cover Test:		Sl esop	Ortho
N.P.C.:		1 in./3 in. OS out; no diplopia	
Retinoscopy/	OD:	–1.75 –1.25 × 21	
Autorefractor:	OS:	–2.00 –1.50 ×175	
Subjective:	OD:	–1.75 –1.25 × 20	VA 20/20 (6/6)
	OS:	–2.00 –1.50 × 175	VA 20/20 (6/6)
Phoria:		Ortho	3 Exop
Base-in vergences:		N/E	X/16/12
Base-out vergences:		N/E	X/18/10
Accom. Amplitude:		4.50	
Neg. Rel. Accom.:		+2.25	
Pos. Rel. Accom.:		–1.25	
Fused X-Cyl.:		+0.50	
Stereo:		N/E	

Assessment

Incipient presbyopia with decreasing myopia.

Plan

We prescribed JW's subjective refraction as a single-vision prescription. He is pleased with the clarity at distance and near through this power. There seems little room for considering any other alternative in this case. JW is pleased he still can avoid a multifocal prescription and asks if he could expect his myopia to continue lessening. We advised that, although it seemed this was the trend, he could not count on his myopia naturally reducing each year. However, to the extent that pseudomyopic accommodative excess can "unravel" in early presbyopia, JW indeed may experience some further reduction in his distance refraction. When he returns next year, we will see whether he can accept further reduction in his spherical or astigmatic minus lens power at distance.

JW experienced a reduction in myopia in the early phases of presbyopia. Other patients with incipient presbyopia may still be susceptible to near-work-induced myopia. This apparently is the case with patients BT and DZ, whose refractive paths follow a different course than JW's.

Subjective

Case History, Including Signs, Symptoms, and Visual Needs

BT is a 50-year-old public school administrator who was first seen in our office 11 years ago. Through the years, her examinations have been unremarkable and her myopia very stable. BT reports that she finds herself taking off her glasses more and more, particularly when meeting with people in her office. She finds this surprising because her friends rely on wearing glasses more frequently. BT also confided that, although age never really concerned her, turning 50 recently gave her pause to reflect on her eye health. She has one sibling, a brother, who has diabetes and experienced a cataract in one eye in his forties that required extraction. He also has been diagnosed with glaucoma, for which he takes medication. Her mother also has glaucoma, which has been treated medically as well as surgically.

Lensometry
OD: −1.50 sphere
OS: −2.25 −0.75 × 175

Objective

Ocular Health Assessment

Automated visual field screening, intraocular pressures, anterior segment, gonioscopic evaluation, and neuroretinal evaluation all are normal.

Clinical Measures

| *Retinoscopy/* | OD: −1.50 sphere | VA 20/20 (6/6) |
| *Autorefractor:* | OS: −2.25 −0.50 × 165 | VA 20/20 (6/6) |

In view of BT's family ocular history, we direct most of our attention to her ocular health, which proves normal. We consider near-point data unessential, as she is pleased with her ability to read simply by removing her glasses. Irrespective of what we would have found, we would not have changed her prescription. We reissue her distance prescription and address her concern about why she is removing her glasses for reading more often. We explain that removing her glasses provides the magnification her friends experience when they put on reading glasses or look through their multifocals. Without her glasses on, the right eye focuses comfortably for computer viewing distances, and her left eye can focus on smaller print at near.

Some patients with eye health concerns jump to the conclusion that any change in visual function may be linked to an eye health problem. In BT's case, it is important to review the results with her to assuage her concerns. BT's ability to adapt to presbyopia by simply removing her myopic prescription for near tasks stands in contrast to her astigmatic counterpart, patient DZ.

Subjective

Case History, Including Signs, Symptoms, and Visual Needs
DZ is a 40-year-old computer analyst for a large regional power company in our area. His general health is excellent, but he has been noticing some variability in his distance vision. At certain times, particularly when driving home from work, it seems more difficult to focus clearly. He wears progressive addition lenses that we initially prescribed 2 years ago and feels comfortable with them for near work. He had done some eye exercises years ago and was concerned about the need to resume them.

Lensometry
OD: −0.25 −1.50 × 11/+1.50
OS: −0.50 −1.50 × 160/+1.50

Objective

Ocular Health Assessment

Internal and external eye structures are healthy and normal in appearance.

Clinical Measures

		At 20 ft (6 m)	*At 16 in. (40 cm)*
VA (cc):	OD:	20/20 (6/6)	20/20 (6/6)
	OS:	20/20 (6/6)	20/20 (6/6)
Cover Test:		X (T)	Ortho
N.P.C.:		2 in./4 in. (5 cm/10 cm) OS out; no diplopia	
Retinoscopy/		Manifest autorefraction,	
Autorefractor:	OD:	−1.25 −2.00 × 5 (8)	
		−0.75 −2.25 × 3 (8)	
		Plano −2.00 × 9 (9)	
	OS:	−1.25 −1.75 × 170 (7)	
		−0.50 −2.00 × 159 (9)	
		Plano −1.75 × 160 (9)	
Subjective:	OD:	−0.25 −1.50 × 10	VA 20/20 (6/6)
	OS:	−0.50 −1.50 × 160	VA 20/20 (6/6)
Phoria:		8 Exop	2 Exop
Base-in vergences:		X/12/8	X/14/12
Base-out vergences:		X/12/6	X/18/14
Accom. Amplitude:		5.50	
Neg. Rel. Accom.:		+2.25	
Pos. Rel. Accom.:		−0.75	
Fused X-Cyl.:		+1.50	
Stereo:		40 seconds of arc	

Assessment

We find DZ has early presbyopia, with divergence excess and secondary accommodative excess resulting in variable, blurred distance vision. Note that we did not administer a cycloplegic refraction, because DZ's fluctuation on manifest autorefraction is sufficiently diagnostic of his condition. Further, he already had been managed effectively by an add so the decision to prescribe plus at near would not have been aided by cycloplegia. Note that DZ does not have the luxury of removing his glasses to obtain clarity at near. Even though he has a spherical equivalent in his distance prescription of –1.00 OD and –1.25 OS, the uncompensated astigmatism induces enough blur that he is more comfortable with an add than removing his glasses for near.

Plan

1. DZ is between a refractive rock and a hard place. He apparently uses some accommodative convergence at distance to maintain fusion. The excess accommodation helps lessen the exodeviation.

2. The progressive addition lens helps DZ relax his excessive accommodation when looking at near, and near point remains comfortable. Therefore, we do not want to fiddle with the net near prescription.

3. We offer DZ the possibility of changing his prescription or engaging in vision therapy. DZ decides to hold off on making any changes in prescription or treatment. As it turns out, his distance findings stabilize without treatment to the point where he is largely asymptomatic.

4. If DZ's symptoms persisted, what would we have done? We could have increased his distance minus by 0.25 sphere OU and offset that with an increase in the add by 0.25 OU. Although this amounts to refractive tweaking, it works in some cases. Another possibility, either in conjunction with increasing minus or independent of it, would be to prescribe a low amount of base-in prism to relieve some of the need to use accommodative convergence at distance. That is more complicated because DZ does not need the prism at near. From previous conversations we know that he would be resistant to using two single-vision prescriptions, one for distance with prism, and one for near without prism. The option to fine tune DZ's accommodative convergence by increasing his base-out vergence range at distance and decreasing the accommodative excess also exists.

Considerations in Adapting to New Eyewear

As discussed in Chapter 5, patients adapting to new eyewear may have difficulty for a variety of reasons, many of which center around changes in spatial perception (Table 3-7). The first and most obvious consideration is the change in image size when a significant increase in myopic lens power occurs. For a child, this can produce almost a fun-house mirror effect. Image size is smaller with higher minus lens power and the brain therefore initially interprets objects as being further away. This holds true even with known relationships, such as the distance from one's eyes to the ground. In addition to the affect on central vision, the quality of peripheral vision decreases as the lens thickness increases. Second, depending on the patient's AC/A ratio, getting adjusted to a higher minus lens value requires some readjustment in binocular vision, which usually occurs rapidly as well. Whenever a significant increase in power is prescribed, patients should be advised that things may look or feel slightly peculiar at first but will adapt within a few days.

More than ever, patients with myopia have a wide selection of lens material and eyewear design. The most cosmetically appealing material to use for higher minus lens prescriptions is high-index glass. When cosmetic appearance is paramount to the patient, we educate him or her about the possibility of using Zeiss high-index glass, which can be fabricated in a center thickness of 1.0 mm. Glass is heavier than high-index plastic or polycarbonate

Table 3-7   Checklist for Adaptive Difficulties

___ Change in lens power or binocularity

___ Change in lens material or index of refraction

___ Change in base curve or asphericity

___ Peripheral lens distortion or warp

___ Change in frame shape or size

___ Position of optical centers

___ Change in pantoscopic angle or faceform fit of frame

___ Change in monocular or binocular interpupillary distance for any given power but provides the most aesthetic edge thickness and appearance. There are medicolegal implications, as the laboratory requires that the doctor sign a waiver on the thinness and the practitioner should have the patient sign a waiver as well, due to the increased possibility of lens shatter on impact.

Generally speaking, the higher is the index of refraction, the thinner the lens edge will be in a given power. However, polycarbonate material is unique in that it can be ground relatively thin at the edges, with minimal center thickness, because of its inherent durability. For most ranges of myopia, a polycarbonate material with a 1.0 mm center thickness provides a cosmetically pleasing result. The earlier versions of polycarbonate tended to result in a birefringence effect that was noticeable as a blue-yellow fringe at the edge of light sources, particularly around fluorescent lights. High index plastic is available in hyperindices with index of refraction as high as 1.74, at this time.

With any lens material, there is a direct correlation between decentration and edge thickness of the lens. In a given power, as decentration values increase, the edge thickness increases. Whenever possible, try to minimize the decentration value, which is the difference between the interpupillary distance (PD) specified to the lab and the mechanical PD (MPD) of the frame. The MPD of the frame is calculated by adding the bridge size to the eye size. The PD normally is the measured anatomical distance between the center of the pupils. Let us take a specific example. Assume that you indicate a PD of 58 and the frame MPD is an eye size 50 with a bridge size of 18, for a total MPD of 68. The decentration value is 10 mm divided by 2, or 5 mm inward for each eye. To help minimize edge thickness, consider increasing the patient's PD if, in your professional judgment, the patient can tolerate the induced prismatic effect. What do we mean by that?

Using Prentice's rule as a guide, each centimeter of decentration induces 1 diopter of prism power per lens power in the horizontal meridian. For minus lenses, lessening the decentration results in a relative base-in prism effect.

We take as a specific example a patient whose habitual prescription is –5.00 sph OU and for whom lensometry shows a PD of 58 mm. Assume that the patient's prescription has not changed, but the patient is electing to get new eyewear. If we use the preceding example and our target value for decentration is 0 for a frame MPD of 68 mm, we would be moving the PD outward by a total of 10 mm from the habitual PD. For a power of –5.00 in the horizontal meridian, the result in this case is a change of 5 prism diopters base in, to which the patient must adapt.

Frame size and shape significantly influence lens edge thickness. For any given lens power and material, the edge thickness increases dramatically as frame size increases and the shape becomes more asymmetrical. To minimize edge thickness, patients with significant amounts of myopia are guided not only to high-index materials with thin centers but relatively small, round frames. Given the propensity of frame manufacturers to alter frame styles, sizes, and shapes in line with fashion industry cycles, clinicians must anticipate the extent to which a patient's adaptive difficulty is related to the resultant change in spatial perception from a change in frame shape or size. High myopes may report that any significant change in frame size or shape results in a "fish bowl" or similar curvature of field perception induced by any of the factors in Table 3-7. Although we advise the patient that it may take a week or two to adapt, some patients will be unwilling to try.

Even though it is not well established that higher amounts of myopia reflect any specific personality type, it would seem wise to take precautions with patients whom you suspect to be visually sensitive.[42] These are patients with whom you have had either prior experience regarding adaptive difficulties or who, during the subjective refraction, are very exacting. By *exacting*, we mean the patient notices a size change in the letters on the chart when you modify the power by 0.25 diopter. You might take the precaution of counseling the frame stylist or optician not to make a significant change in any of the variables in Table 3-7 and specify "zero tolerance" on the lab slip. Before the patient is called for dispensing, the individual responsible for verifying completed work from the lab should confirm all information that has been specified, including base curves.

The majority of patients do not require this degree of consideration or specification about ophthalmic variables. They can be

Table 3-8   Optometric Management of the Patient with Myopia

Simple myopia	
Infants/toddlers	Prescription if myopia >3 D
School-age children	Prescription if myopia >1–2 D
Adults	Prescribe to improve DVA
Myopia control	Plus lens add at near, RGPs, visual hygiene
Myopia reduction	Orthokeratology, refractive surgery
Pseudomyopia	
Myopia control	Plus lens add at near, VT, cyclotherapeusis
Night myopia	
Myopia compensation	Additional myopic lens power for night driving
Induced myopia	
Myopia containment	Reduce influence of myopiagenic agent (e.g., stress reduction, nutrition)
Degenerative myopia	
Structural changes	Monitor retina and manage treatment as indicated

Source: Adapted from *Optometric Clinical Practice Guideline: Care of the Patient with Myopia.* St. Louis: American Optometric Association, 1997:63.
DVA, distance visual acuity; RGPs, rigid gas-permeables; VT, vision therapy.

managed through the general guidelines summarized in this chapter (Table 3-8). The few who do occupy the majority of your time in refractive problem solving. Although you can minimize the time spent by anticipating adaptive difficulties in advance, some patients will seem difficult to satisfy. These even may be patients for whom you prescribed successfully in the past but cannot seem to satisfy presently. As we note in Chapter 5, you need to identify the point where you either cannot afford to spend additional time or have simply exhausted all reasonable possibilities to account for the patient's difficulties. At that point, it is wise to arrange some equitable compensation for your time and the patient's troubles and move on.

References

1. Grosvenor T, Goss DA. *Clinical Management of Myopia.* Boston: Butterworth–Heinemann, 1999.

2. Press LJ (ed). *Applied Concepts in Vision Therapy*. St. Louis: Mosby, 1997:21–28.

3. Rosner J, Rosner J. *Pediatric Optometry*, 2nd ed. Boston: Butterworth–Heinemann, 1990:363.

4. Gallop A, Kitchener G. Myopia: An orientation. In: A Barber (ed). *Myopia Control*. Santa Ana, CA: Optometric Extension Program, 1998:1–11.

5. Ong E, Ciuffreda KJ. Accommodation, Nearwork and Myopia. Santa Ana, CA: Optometric Extension Program, 1997.

6. Sherman A, Press LJ. Myopia control: Taming the refractive beast. In: LJ Press (ed). *Applied Concepts in Vision Therapy*. St. Louis: Mosby, 1997:180–187.

7. Birnbaum MH. *Optometric Management of Nearpoint Vision Disorders*. Boston: Butterworth–Heinemann, 1993:11–32, 196–203.

8. Sherman A. Myopia can often be prevented, controlled or eliminated. *J Behav Optom*. 1993;4:16–22.

9. Rosenfield M, Gilmartin B (eds). *Myopia and Nearwork*. Boston: Butterworth–Heinemann, 1998.

10. Thorn F, Troilo D, Gwiazda J (eds). *Myopia 2000: Proceedings of the Eighth International Conference on Myopia*. Boston, July 7–9, 2000.

11. Zadnik K, Mutti Do, Friedman NE, et al. Ocular predictors of the onset of juvenile myopia. *Invest Ophthalmol Vis Sci*. 1999;40:1936–1943.

12. Fulk GW, Cyert LA, Parker DE. A randomized trial on the effect of single-vision lenses vs. bifocal lenses on myopia progression in children with esophoria. *Optom Vis Sci*. 2000; 77:395–401.

13. Goss DA, Grosvenor T. Rates of childhood myopia progression with bifocals as a function of nearpoint phoria: Consistency of three studies. *Optom Vis Sci*. 1990;67:637–640.

14. Press LJ. Control of progressive myopia. In: LJ Press, BD Moore (eds). *Clinical Pediatric Optometry*. Boston: Butterworth–Heinemann, 1993:329–330.

15. Press LJ. Accommodation and vergence disorders: Restoring balance to a distressed system. In: Press LJ (ed). *Applied Concepts in Vision Therapy*. St. Louis: Mosby, 1997:114.

16. Press LJ. Correspondence. *Optom Vis Sci*. 2000;77:630–631.

17. Wick B. On the etiology of refractive error—Part III. *J Optom Vis Devel.* 2000;31:93-99.
18. Birnbaum MH. *Optometric Management of Nearpoint Vision Disorder.* Boston: Butterworth–Heinemann, 1993:162–163.
19. Goss DA, Uyesugi EF. Effectiveness of bifocal control of childhood myopia progression as a function of near point phoria and binocular cross-cylinder. *J Optom Vis Devel.* 1995; 26:12–17.
20. Zadnik K, Mutti DO, Friedman NE, et al. Ocular predictors of the onset of juvenile myopia. *Invest Ophthalmol Vis Sci.* 1999;40:1936–1943.
21. Press LJ. Students with persistent problems: The visual connection. *School Nurse News.* 2000;17(4):38–39.
22. Foerster R. On the influence of concave glasses and convergence of the ocular axes in the increase of myopia. *Arch Ophthalmol.* 1886;15:399–435.
23. Birnbaum MH. Management of the low myopia pediatric patient. *J Am Optom Assoc.* 1979;50:1281–1289.
24. Ebenholtz SM. Accommodative hysteresis: A precursor to induced myopia? *Invest Ophthalmol Vis Sci.* 1983;24:513–515.
25. Bullimore MA, Gilmartin B. Aspects of tonic accommodation in late onset myopia. *Am J Optom Physiol Opt.* 1987;64: 499–503.
26. Ciuffreda KJ, Ordonez X. Vision therapy to reduce abnormal nearwork-induced transient myopia. *Optom Vis Sci.* 1998;75: 311–315.
27. Hung GK, Ciuffreda KJ. Adaptation model of nearwork-induced transient myopia. *Ophthal Physiol Optics.* 1999;19: 151–158.
28. Hung GK, Ciuffreda KJ. A unifying theory of refractive error development. *Bull Math Biol.* 2000;3:1–21.
29. Press LJ. Topical review of the literature: Myopia. *J Optom Vis Devel.* 1987;18:1–17.
30. Press LJ. Topical review of the literature: Lenses and behavior. *J Optom Vis Devel.* 1990;21:5–17.
31. Goss DA. *Ocular Accommodation, Convergence, and Fixation Disparity: A Manual of Clinical Analysis,* 2nd ed. Boston: Butterworth–Heinemann, 1995.

32. Scheiman M, Wick B. *Clinical Management of Binocular Vision.* Philadelphia: Lippincott, 1994:41–42.
33. Ong E, Ciuffreda KJ. *Accommodation, Nearwork and Myopia.* Santa Ana, CA: Optometric Extension Program, 1997:134–135.
34. Manas L. *Visual Analysis Handbook.* Chicago: Professional Press, 1952:30.
35. Rutstein RP. Daum KM, Amos JF. Accommodative spasm: A study of 17 cases. *J Am Optom Assoc.* 1988;59:527–538.
36. Forrest EB. *Stress and Vision.* Santa Ana, CA: Optometric Extension Program, 1988:176.
37. Jacques L. Dad's point of view. *Optometric Monthly.* October 1979:689–692.
38. Sherman A, Press LJ. Myopia control therapy. In: LJ Press (ed). *Applied Concepts in Vision Therapy.* St. Louis: Mosby, 1997:306.
39. Bartlett JD, Jaanus JD. *Clinical Ocular Pharmacology,* 4th ed. Boston: Butterworth–Heinemann, 2001:919.
40. Mahoney BP, Cavallerano J. Systemic considerations and ocular manifestations of diabetes mellitus. In: Muchnick BG. *Clinical Medicine in Optometric Practice.* St. Louis: Mosby, 1994: 275–276.
41. Ciuffreda KJ. Accommodation, the pupil, and presbyopia. In: Benjamin WB (ed). *Borish's Clinical Refraction.* Philadelphia: Saunders, 1998:109.
42. Lanyon RI, Giddings JW. Psychological approaches to myopia: A review. *Am J Optom Physiol Opt.* 1974;51:271–281.

CHAPTER 4

Prescribing for the Patient with Hyperopia

The decision to prescribe lenses for a patient with hyperopia and the amount of lens power prescribed depend on a number of interrelated factors. Rather than intersperse case examples of prescribing lenses for patients with hyperopia, we identify some general principles first and then devote a separate section to case examples. In contrast with myopia, the patient with a moderate amount of hyperopia rarely complains of blur until presbyopia emerges. However, visual fatigue or discomfort may ensue when the patient has accommodative insufficiency at any age and warrants prescribing even for low amounts of hyperopia.[1] Moderate to high amounts of hyperopia also warrant a lens prescription in the absence of blur when fusional divergence ability is poor and the accommodative effort to compensate for the hyperopia results in excessive esophoria or in esotropia.[2] Uncorrected hyperopia also has been shown to be associated with a higher prevalence of substandard visual perceptual and reading abilities.[3,4]

Classification of Hyperopia

The terminology associated with hyperopia, and particularly regarding cycloplegic refraction and prescribing, can be confusing. In proof, optometric clinicians rarely speak in textbook terms of absolute, facultative, relative, or total hyperopia. We offer the following streamlined definitions, which are relevant to our case discussions:

- *Manifest hyperopia* is the amount of hyperopia derived through noncycloplegic ("dry") refraction.
- *Total hyperopia* is the amount of hyperopia derived through cycloplegic ("wet") refraction.
- *Latent hyperopia* is the difference between noncycloplegic and cycloplegic refraction.
- *Absolute hyperopia* is the amount of hyperopia that cannot be compensated for by accommodation.

Manifest hyperopia is indicated by the maximum plus lens that provides the optimum distance visual acuity.[5] The relaxation of accommodation at distance to reveal maximum hyperopia in routine refraction is accomplished through a reduction in the stimulus to accommodation with added convex lens power.[6] Technically speaking, some degree of latent hyperopia can be revealed on a delayed subjective refraction by inducing the patient to relax accommodation through more than the usual amount of plus lens "fog" at distance. However, the full amount of latent hyperopia is determined through a reduction in the response to accommodation, best accomplished through cycloplegic pharmaceutical agents.

Cycloplegic Refraction

There are numerous reasons for conducting a cycloplegic refraction (Table 4-1). The goal in all instances is to elicit the maximum amount of hyperopia. This not only helps the clinician gain a more complete picture of the patient's visual profile but can be a useful aid in prescribing lenses. In all instances, a manifest ("dry") refraction should be conducted prior to the installation of cycloplegic agents. Amos suggests a preinstallation ocular health evaluation, which follows the same precautions as one would consider prior to pupillary dilation.[7]

The standard topical pharmaceutical agent for cycloplegic refraction is 1% cyclopentolate. Following instillation of topical

Table 4-1   Indications for Cycloplegic Refraction

Suspected latent hyperopia

Suspected pseudomyopia

Accommodative esophoria

Accommodative esotropia

Variable retinoscopic or autorefractor findings

Variable subjective findings during "dry" refraction

Visual acuity not correctable to expected levels

Symptoms seemingly unrelated to manifest refraction

Source: Adapted from Amos JF. Cycloplegic refraction. In: JD
Bartlett, SD Jaanus (eds). *Clinical Ocular Pharmacology*, 4th ed.
Boston: Butterworth–Heinemann, 2001:426.

anesthetic, 2 drops of 1% cyclopentolate are instilled, with 5 minutes allowed between drops.[8] Although 1 drop of 1% cyclopentolate may be inadequate for patients with dark brown irides,[9] we often find that 1 drop is adequate for patients with lightly pigmented irides. The peak of cycloplegia with 1% cyclopentolate can be attained in as little as 25 minutes,[10] and typically sooner with lightly pigmented patients.

As a matter of protocol, we have an assistant readminister the automated refractor after 20 minutes for each patient. Any significant change in refraction should be evident as a hyperopic shift of at least 0.50 diopter after 20 minutes. In other words, if latent hyperopia can be unmasked relatively quickly with 1 drop of 1% cyclopentolate, consider prescribing more plus than the patient normally accepts on dry refraction. However, latent hyperopia revealed only after 2 drops of 1% cyclopentolate and at a duration of 45 minutes or more is unlikely to be accepted by the patient if included in the lens prescription. We elaborate on this in the next section and through one of the case examples.

The Acceptance of Plus Lens Prescriptions

Most clinicians agree that a distance lens prescription is not indicated for low amounts of hyperopia. In fact, as noted by Birnbaum, Skeffington postulated that low hyperopia is an advantageous state that serves as a buffer against the development of myopia.[11] In our case discussions in this chapter, we do not treat hyperopia as an adaptive response, although readers interested in this perspective are encouraged to avail themselves of Birnbaum's text for the many references to functional viewpoints on hyperopia and other refractive states. However, we do adopt the OEP (Optometric Extension Program) philosophy of being conservative about the amount of plus prescribed for distance (Table 4-2).

OEP case types, based on the interrelationship of accommodation and vergence findings as compared to expected values, were formulated in part to predict the acceptability of plus lens prescriptions. As related by Manas, the hyperopic lens value prescribed for the patient usually is less that the subjective refraction except in the B-1 case type, where full plus can be prescribed at distance.[12] Our case examples do not go through OEP analysis or case typing, but **clinical pearl 7** emphasizes the importance of being conservative in the amount of plus lens power prescribed for distance. The patient may complain of blur or a generalized feeling of the prescription not being correct when the amount of plus at distance is increased by as little as +0.25 or +0.50 diopter.

Every experienced clinician learns early in his or her career that some patients with low to moderate amounts of hyperopia are happier without a lens prescription, particularly at distance, even if there is a slight increase in visual acuity. The same holds true of patients with moderate to high amounts of hyperopia who are happier with considerably less than their full distance subjec-

Table 4-2   Distance Prescription Guidelines in Latent Hyperopia

	Cycloplegic Refraction		
Manifest Refraction	*1.00*	*2.50*	*5.00*
Plano	0.50	1.00	2.00
1.00	1.00	1.50	2.25
2.00	N/A	2.25	2.75
3.00	N/A	N/A	3.75

tive refraction. Blur is not a reliable determinant of how well the patient is going to respond to the plus lens power at distance. Inability to adapt to the prescription rarely is predicted by clarity alone or results of the bichrome balance test. A patient may note that, through the phoropter, the full plus lens power on subjective refraction makes the letters look larger or easier to see. However, when the patient is trial framed, the distance subjective may result in a feeling of discomfort or even mild postural imbalance or nausea. This is particularly true when the patient does not habitually wear a distance lens prescription.

If we decide to reduce the amount of plus prescribed at distance, particularly when there is a range of power through which the patient cannot discern much difference in clarity or comfort, the amount of plus prescribed tends to be arbitrary.[13] This is true particularly with the patient's first lens prescription. When the patient is symptomatic and experiences esophoria, one guideline is to prescribe the minimum amount of plus that reduces the esophoria to orthophoria. In general, prescribe the least amount of plus that results in subjective improvement of either distance acuity or comfort, while the patient is walking around the office or looking at distance signage through the tentative prescription.

In summary, factors that influence the patient's satisfaction with hyperopic lens prescriptions include the amount of ametropia; the patient's age, visual needs, and experience with prior lens prescriptions; the influence of prescribing on the accommodative and vergence systems; and the patient's overall visual performance and sensitivity. For young children, the importance of an appropriate plus lens prescription on accommodative esotropia is widely recognized. However, the timing of an appropriate lens prescription also can have profound effects on a child's visual perceptual development.[14]

Adapting to Changes in Lens Prescription

In the previous section, we allude to potential adaptation difficulties in changing lens prescriptions. Factors relating to induced spatial distortion and subsequent adaptive strategies are elaborated in the chapters on myopia and astigmatism. Another factor relates to all prescription changes yet is distinct from traditional considerations of binocular vision and spatial localization: the adaptive learning required in the VOR (vestibuloocular reflex) each time a change in lens prescription occurs. It, in essence, is a dynamic reorganization of the relationship between space and time mediated through the visual system.

The VOR stabilizes the image of the visual world, transmitted through the retina, from appearing to move during passive or active movements of the head. Unlike accommodation/vergence interaction, the VOR is an open loop reflex that operates without the benefit of immediate sensory feedback. The synaptic connections between the vestibular ganglion cells and the motor neurons of the extraocular muscles are calibrated based on experience and represents a form of learning.

Learning in the VOR system has been demonstrated in experiments in which an observer wears lenses that change magnification, creating a mismatch between eye movements produced by the VOR and the amount of movement required to keep the image in place based on local retinal changes.[15] For example, without glasses, a rotation of the head to the right at 10° per second requires movements of the eyes to the left at 10° per second. When a lens prescription is given that increases magnification, the light spread function at the retinal level is of an image that is larger than what previously had been calibrated. As a result, rotation of the head at 10° per second now produces movement of the image on the retina at greater than 10° per second. When the VOR produces the previously correct eye movements at 10° per second, the motion of the eyes is insufficient to correct the slippage of the image on the retina, and the visual world appears to move to the left as the head rotates to the right.

The patient who successfully adapts to the increase in magnification induced by the change in plus lens power has learned to increase the output of the VOR so that the retinal image once again is stabilized while the head rotates. The change in VOR can be expressed in terms of the gain of the reflex, specifically the relation between head rotation (input velocity) and eye rotation (output velocity). When input equals output and the gain is 1.0, no motion is perceived as the eyes move. With an increase in plus lens power, the gain initially is greater than 1.0; with a decrease in plus lens power, the gain initially is less than 1.0. The cerebellum plays an important role in adjusting the gain of the VOR to minimize image motion during head rotation. This is one reason why we suggest to patients who obtain new glasses with which we anticipate adaptive difficulty or to patients who complain of adaptive difficulty to initially use the new prescription in familiar surroundings. As the patients adjust, we encourage full-time wear of the prescription and tell them to hide their previous glasses, so that VOR recalibration is reinforced through cerebellar learning under a variety of movement conditions.

Case Examples

Subjective

Case History, Including Signs, Symptoms, and Visual Needs
Patient KB, a 6-year-old child, presents for her first comprehensive eye examination. We previously examined her parents and older sister, none of whom wear glasses. She has no visual complaints and is considered by her teacher to be a model student. Her parents report that she is bright and loves to read.

Lensometry
No prior prescription.

Objective

Ocular Health Assessment
N/E

Clinical Measures

	At 20 ft (6 m)	At 16 in. (40 cm)
VA (unaided):	OD: 20/20 (6/6)	20/20 (6/6)
	OS: 20/20 (6/6)	20/20 (6/6)
Cover Test:	Ortho	Sl exop
N.P.C.:	To the nose	
Retinoscopy/	OD: +0.75 –0.25 × 10	
Autorefractor:	OS: +0.75 –0.25 × 170	

	At 20 ft (6 m)	*At 16 in. (40 cm)*
Subjective:	OD: +0.50 sphere	VA 20/20 (6/6)
	OS: +0.50 sphere	VA 20/20 (6/6)
Phoria:	1 exop	5 exop
Base-in vergences:	N/E	N/E
Base-out vergences:	N/E	N/E
Accom. Amplitude:	N/E	
Neg. Rel. Accom.:	N/E	
Pos. Rel. Accom.:	N/E	
Fused X-Cyl.:	+0.25	
Stereo:	20 seconds of arc	

Assessment

Low hyperopia OU.

Plan

There is no indication to give KB a lens prescription from a classical point of view. KB's school performance is excellent and she enjoys reading. One might consider conducting other forms of retinoscopy or performance tests to assess indications for low power plus lenses at near.

Subjective

Case History, Including Signs, Symptoms, and Visual Needs

Patient HL, an 8-year-old child, presents for her first comprehensive eye examination. We have not examined any of her family members, but neither of her parents wears glasses and she is an only child. HL is struggling in school. Although she comprehends well when listening, she has a lot of difficulty when trying to read independently. She reports that, when she "lets her eyes loose," the words get blurry. Her parents took her to an eye doctor last year who advised that although HL is mildly farsighted, glasses were not indicated.

Lensometry

No prior prescription.

Objective

Ocular Health Assessment

N/E

Clinical Measures

		At 20 ft (6 m)	*At 16 in. (40 cm)*
VA (unaided):	OD:	20/20 (6/6)	20/20 (6/6)
	OS:	20/20 (6/6)	20/20 (6/6)
Cover Test:		Ortho	Sl esop
N.P.C.:		To the nose	
Retinoscopy/	OD:	+1.00 –0.25 × 180	
Autorefractor:	OS:	+1.00 –0.25 × 180	
Subjective:	OD:	+075 sphere	VA 20/20 (6/6)
	OS:	+0.75 sphere	VA 20/20 (6/6)
Phoria:		Ortho	2 exop
Base-in vergences:		N/E	8/12/6
Base-out vergences:		N/E	X/24/18
Accom. Amplitude:		10 diopters	
Neg. Rel. Accom.:		+2.00	
Pos. Rel. Accom.:		–1.75	
Fused X-Cyl.:		+0.50	
Stereo:		20 seconds of arc	

Assessment

Low hyperopia OU.

Plan

Because of her symptoms and performance difficulties in reading, we decide to give HL a low plus lens prescription. HL's binocular profile looks well balanced at near through the subjective refraction, particularly the shift from low esophoria unaided to low exophoria through the lenses. A single-vision power of +0.75 sph OU was trial framed and well accepted. The single-vision lens is primarily for reading but does not blur distance vision as when copying from the blackboard.

Subjective

Case History, Including Signs, Symptoms, and Visual Needs

Patient AC, a 7-year-old child, has not been examined previously. She is an outspoken child, who is generally in good health and takes Claritin daily. Her mother reports that AC tends to misidentify letters and skips lines when reading. AC had a very difficult time learning in school last year, and her mother has home schooled her this year. AC has a 5-year-old sister who has no difficulties with learning.

Lensometry

No prior prescription.

Objective

Ocular Health Assessment

N/E

Clinical Measures

		At 20 ft (6 m)	At 16 in. (40 cm)
VA (unaided):	OD:	20/20 (6/6)	20/20 (6/6)
	OS:	20/20 (6/6)	20/20 (6/6)
Cover Test:		Ortho	4 esop
N.P.C.:		To the nose	
Manifest Retinoscopy/	OD:	+0.25 –0.25 × 90	
Autorefractor:	OS:	Plano	
Manifest Subjective:	OD:	Plano	VA 20/20 (6/6)
	OS:	Plano	VA 20/20 (6/6)
Phoria:		Ortho	3 esop
Base-in vergences:		N/E	X/10/2
Base-out vergences:		N/E	X/20/18
Accom. Amplitude:		11 diopters	
Neg. Rel. Accom.:		+1.50	
Pos. Rel. Accom.:		–2.00	
Fused X-Cyl.:		+0.25	
Stereo:		40 seconds of arc	
MEM Retinoscopy:		+0.25 lag OU	

Cycloplegic	OD: +1.25 –0.25 × 175	
Retinoscopy/	OS: +1.50 –0.25 × 10	
Autorefractor:		
Manifest Subjective:	OD: +1.25	VA 20/20 (6/6)
	OS: +1.25	VA 20/20 (6/6)

Assessment

Latent hyperopia OU.

Plan

We prescribed a multifocal lens with a power of plano/+1.00 OU.

1. There are alternative ways to manage AC's case. Since she is home schooled, seeing the blackboard clearly across the room is not an issue. So at least for this school year, we could have given her a single-vision lens. However, giving a child a bifocal lens also affords some passive accommodative rock therapy whenever she looks up, whether to mother's face or something that mother might be demonstrating, even a few feet away.

2. If there is esophoria at near, and particularly when there are learning problems, a plus lens prescription is strongly indicated. Even though conventional findings in this case provide no guidance for how much plus at near to prescribe, the difference between the manifest (dry) and latent (wet) refraction provides an acceptable indication of the maximum amount of plus to prescribe initially at near. This is illustrated in Table 4-3.

Table 4-3   Guideline for Add Calculation in Latent Hyperopia

Add power = cycloplegic refraction – manifest refraction	
Example:	Cycloplegic refraction = +3.00
	Manifest refraction = +1.25
	Add value = +1.75
	Final prescription = +1.25/+1.75

Subjective

Case History, Including Signs, Symptoms, and Visual Needs

Patient AV, a 31-year-old homemaker, recalls having glasses prescribed for her as a young child, but never wearing them. She is beginning to work out of her home, which involves using a computer, and finds it difficult to maintain focus. She notices that after she finishes doing near work, there is some delay in being able to refocus to distance. This has made her more sensitive to some blur when watching television. AV is a sports fan, and the boxed scores in the corner of the screen are getting harder to read.

AV takes no medication other than self-selected herbal extracts and supplements, and her general health is reportedly excellent. She went for an eye examination a few months ago and was given prescription lenses that she could not wear comfortably. AV told the eye doctor that she could see okay, but the lenses felt too strong and she was more comfortable without them. He advised her that she would get used to them. When AV mentioned her difficulties to her neighbor, a patient of ours, the neighbor recommended she come to our office.

Lensometry
OD: +2.25 –0.50 × 130
OS: +1.50 sphere

Objective

Ocular Health Assessment
N/E

Clinical Measures

	At 20 ft (6 m)	At 16 in. (40 cm)
VA (unaided):	OD: 20/25 (6/7.5)	20/25 (6/7.5)
	OS: 20/20 (6/6)	20/20 (6/6)
Cover Test:	Ortho	
N.P.C.:	To the nose	
Retinoscopy/	OD: +2.50 –1.00 × 128	
Autorefractor:	OS: +1.50 –0.25 × 180	

	At 20 ft (6 m)	*At 16 in. (40 cm)*
Subjective:	OD: +2.00 −1.00 × 135	VA 20/20 (6/6)
	OS: +1.50 sphere	VA 20/20 (6/6)
Phoria:	1 exop	4 exop
Base-in vergences:	N/E	X/16/10
Base-out vergences:	N/E	X/22/18
Accom. Amplitude:	6 diopters	
Neg. Rel. Accom.:	+1.75	
Pos. Rel. Accom.:	−1.75	
Fused X-Cyl.:	Plano	
Stereo:	40 seconds of arc	

Assessment

Moderate hyperopia OU.

Plan

We prescribe a single-vision lens prescription of +1.00 sph OU to be used for all near-point activity and optionally for television viewing when tired. A few days after she received the eyewear, we call AV to she how she is doing. She is delighted with the comfort as well as clarity of the glasses and is using them as we had suggested.

1. Because AV never wore the glasses prescribed for her as a child, we can consider this her first lens prescription in anticipating adaptation issues.
2. The previous doctor prescribed the full subjective refraction, which was more than what is required to address the patient's needs. Several clinical pearls are violated here. **Clinical pearl 7** cautions against prescribing too much plus at distance. Trial framing with the patient looking beyond the confines of the examination room is the best way to tell if the tentative prescription has too much plus lens power. We can use a sign at the end of a long hallway or viewing street signs out a window. In addition, as noted in **clinical pearl 8**, when there is a change from the habitual state of more than 1 diopter, it is wise to prescribe the change in stages. Following

this advice also leads to less plus than the previous doctor prescribed.

3. We elect to drop the cylinder from the prescription, given that AV's reduction in accommodation was the principal factor in her symptoms. We also prefer to make symmetrical lens changes from the habitual state whenever possible, as mentioned in **clinical pearl 6**.

Subjective

Case History, Including Signs, Symptoms, and Visual Needs

Patient SM, a 32-year-old buyer, is a full-time soft contact lens wearer who reports having esotropia as a child but grew out of it. We were unable to document this with past records, but SM volunteered that she always had slightly better vision with her right eye than her left. She has a history of iritis, treated successfully 2 years ago with topical steroids. She has been using +1.50 over-the-counter readers successfully in conjunction with her contact lenses for the past five years. SM wears daily wear disposable lenses, with a power of +3.50 OD and +3.25 OS and believes this to be the same power she has in her glasses. She can interchange between contact lenses and glasses with no problem.

Lensometry
OD: +3.50
OS: +3.25

Objective

Ocular Health Assessment

Anterior chambers white and quiet OU, with no cells or flare. Mild giant pupillary conjunctivitis (GPC), but otherwise all external and internal eye health findings normal.

Clinical Measures

	At 20 ft (6 m)	At 16 in. (40 cm)
VA (aided):	OD: 20/20 (6/6)	20/25 (6/7.5)
	OS: 20/20 (6/6)	20/25 (6/7.5)
Cover Test:	Sl esop	Sl esop

	At 20 ft (6 m)	*At 16 in. (40 cm)*
N.P.C.:	To the nose	
Retinoscopy/	OD: +3.50 –0.50 × 110	
Autorefractor:	OS: +3.50 –0.50 × 85	
Subjective:	OD: +3.50 –0.50 × 105	VA 20/20
	OS: +3.50 –0.50 × 90	VA 20/25
Phoria:	2 esop	4 esop
Phoria through +1.50 add:		Ortho
Base-in vergences:	N/E	X/8/4
Phoria through +1.50 add:		X/14/12
Base-out vergences:	N/E	N/E
Accom. Amplitude:	5 diopters	
Neg. Rel. Accom.:	+2.50	
Pos. Rel. Accom.:	Plano	
Fused X-Cyl.:	+1.75	
Stereo:	100 seconds of arc	

Assessment

Appreciable hyperopia OU with accommodative insufficiency.

Plan

Clinical pearl 14 is operative here: It is hard to improve on an asymptomatic state.

We educate SM about accommodation and convergence issues in lay terms and reissued the same spectacle and contact lenses as she wears habitually. Because she is well adapted to her current prescription and has no binocular or performance difficulties, we agree that there is no indication for further treatment. There is the distinct possibility that SM's binocular vision would decompensate in the future, and she indicates interest in considering treatment in the future.

Subjective

Case History, Including Signs, Symptoms, and Visual Needs

Patient AS, a 27-year-old artist, received her first plus lens prescription from us 5 years ago. At that time she was experiencing a lot of visual stress and her vision seemed to fluctuate a bit. We found that she was a low hyperope and prescribed plus lenses that stabilized her vision. Things have been going smoothly, but she's now helping her father run his store, where a variety of paintings are displayed, and helping mount frames. AS is experiencing a slight recurrence of the fluctuation in vision and eyestrain she had prior to getting glasses, even with the glasses on. She is beginning to feel "tied to her glasses" and is concerned about the prospect of having to use them more often. Her general health has been excellent.

Lensometry
OD: +0.50
OS: +0.50

Objective

Ocular Health Assessment
All findings are normal.

Clinical Measures

	At 20 ft (6 m)	At 16 in. (40 cm)
VA (unaided):	OD: 20/20 (6/6)	20/20 (6/6)
	OS: 20/20 (6/6)	20/20 (6/6)
Cover Test:	Ortho	Ortho
N.P.C.:	To the nose	
Retinoscopy/	OD: +1.25 –0.50 × 124	
Autorefractor:	OS: +1.50 –0.50 × 52	
Subjective:	OD: +1.25 –0.50 × 125	VA 20/20 (6/6)
	OS: +1.25 –0.50 × 50	VA 20/20 (6/6)
Phoria:	Ortho	3 exop
Base-in vergences:	N/E	X/14/10
Base-out vergences:	N/E	X/18/10
Accom. Amplitude:	8 diopters	
Neg. Rel. Accom.:	+2.00	
Pos. Rel. Accom.:	–2.00	
Fused X-Cyl.:	+0.75	
Stereo:	N/E	

Assessment

Low hyperopia with mild increase in hyperopic refraction.

Plan

We increase the lens prescription to +0.75 sphere OU.

1. Note that AS expresses the concern that she does not want to become too reliant on her prescription. Clinical experience tells us that hyperopes who have more plus prescribed than is necessary to meet their needs find themselves more symptomatic when not wearing the glasses than they had been. Clinical experience also predicts that the need for the next increase in prescription will come faster when the maximum acceptable plus is prescribed for the hyperope as opposed to the minimum amount of plus necessary.

2. **Clinical pearl 9** cautions that a 0.25 diopter lens change rarely addresses asthenopic symptoms satisfactorily, with the exception of presbyopia and visually sensitive patients. As an artist, AS certainly fits into the latter category. We suggest in **clinical pearl 9** that trial framing the patients in such cases and telling them what they might expect from the change in lenses is critical. AS appreciates that +0.25 sph OU over her habitual +0.50 sph OU makes things feel more comfortable. When we trial frame the full subjective refraction, AS reports feeling disoriented and even a bit nauseous. We reduce the power to +1.00 sph OU, the spherical equivalent of the refraction, but AS still comparatively prefers the +0.75 sph OU. It is possible that we could have increased AS's prescription to +1.00 sph OU and she would adapt to the initial sensation. Again, however, we find no virtue in pushing unnecessary amounts of plus.

3. The binocular and accommodative findings show that AS is relatively well balanced, but frankly, we would have prescribed the same lenses irrespective of the binocular findings. There is no need to consider an add, and given AS's feelings about becoming dependent on the glasses, she would likely have rejected the concept. Were AS to feel no

improvement through the new prescription, we would consider the option of vision therapy or prism, particularly if the nonrefractive visual findings are askew.

Subjective

Case History, Including Signs, Symptoms, and Visual Needs

Patient GH, a 38-year-old court stenographer, is a long-standing patient who has been using a near-point lens prescription for the past 10 years. She is in for her yearly comprehensive examination and notes that her health remains excellent and she takes no medications. She is more conscious now of needing to put on her glasses when doing extended close work but still feels fine watching television and driving without glasses.

Lensometry

OD: +1.00 –0.75 × 118
OS: +0.50 –0.50 × 73

Objective

Ocular Health Assessment

All findings are normal.

Clinical Measures

	At 20 ft (6 m)	At 16 in. (40 cm)
VA (unaided):	OD: 20/20 –2 (6/6 –2)	20/30 (6/9)
	OS: 20/20 (6/6)	20/25 (6/7.5)
Cover Test:	Ortho	Sl exop
N.P.C.:	3 in./6 in. (7.5 cm/15 cm) OD out	
Retinoscopy/	OD: +1.50 –1.00 × 120	
Autorefractor:	OS: +1.00 –0.50 × 75	
Subjective:	OD: +1.50 –1.00 × 120	VA 20/20
	OS: +1.00 –0.50 × 75	VA 20/20 (6/6)
Phoria:	1 exop	6 exop
Base-in vergences:	N/E	N/E
Base-out vergences:	N/E	N/E
Accom. Amplitude:	6 diopters	
Neg. Rel. Accom.:	N/E	

Pos. Rel. Accom.:	N/E
Fused X-Cyl.:	+1.50
Stereo:	N/E

Assessment

Low compound hyperopic astigmatism with emerging presbyopia.

Plan

GH wants to select a new frame, and we reissue her habitual lens prescription, adjusting the cylinder axes by a couple of degrees in each eye to match the current subjective.

1. The old standby **clinical pearl 14** is operative here, advising us not to try to improve on the asymptomatic state.
2. The most common mistake in a case of this nature is to observe that the patient can accept more plus lens power at distance than is contained in her current near prescription and to encourage her to increase her lens power. After all, the increased plus lens power not only will be better at near but will not cause blur when looking across the room or walking around.
3. GH is approaching 40 years old. As discussed in Chapter 6, patients at this age are concerned about becoming dependent on glasses for reading. They certainly want to push off using glasses for distance as long as possible. So in general, you do GH no favor by increasing her prescription power in this case. There is the temptation to think that since GH will likely need an increase in plus lens power in a year or two, we should increase it slightly now when she is getting new glasses anyway. Although we will not quibble over increasing the plus sphere by 0.25 in one or both eyes, and GH may accept that increase, it will only heighten her sense of having to rely on the prescription more when glancing at near print.
4. We would advise not to encourage GH to consider a multifocal lens. Some practitioners may be overzealous in wanting to push significantly more plus lens power, but there is

no virtue in this for patient GH because she functions very well at distance without any prescription.

5. Virtually all of the binocular findings are nonessential in this case because we have no intention of altering GH's prescription based on the phorias and vergences. Nor is there any preventive care we would recommend in this case based on changes in GH's binocular profile. Given the luxury of time, additional binocular data may be gathered to round out the clinical picture.

Subjective

Case History, Including Signs, Symptoms, and Visual Needs

Patient DR, a 46-year-old schoolteacher, is a new patient who wears 2-week disposable contact lenses on a monovision basis. Her right lens power is +2.25 and her left lens power is +3.50. DR indicates that her current contact lens prescription meets all her visual needs. However, her spectacle lens prescription has not been changed for awhile. Although she does not wear her glasses often, DR is aware of the need to have a viable alternative to her contact lenses on days when she should take a break from contact lens wear. She wants to rely on our advice about the need to update her habitual progressive spectacle lens power.

Lensometry

OD: +1.75 –0.50 × 92/+1.50
OS: +1.50 sphere/+1.50

Objective

Ocular Health Assessment
All findings are normal.

Clinical Measures

	At 20 ft (6 m)	*At 16 in. (40 cm)*
VA (aided):	OD: 20/25 (6/7.5)	20/25 (6/7.5)
	OS: 20/25 (6/7.5)	20/25 (6/7.5)
Cover Test:	Ortho	Sl exop
N.P.C.:	N/E	

	At 20 ft (6 m)	*At 16 in. (40 cm)*
Retinoscopy/	OD: +3.50 –1.00 × 50	
Autorefractor:	OS: +2.75 –0.50 × 155	
Subjective:	OD: +3.00 –1.00 × 50	VA 20/20 (6/6)
	OS: +2.50 –0.50 × 155	VA 20/20 (6/6)
Phoria:	1 exop	5 exop
Base-in vergences:	N/E	N/E
Base-out vergences:	N/E	N/E
Accom. Amplitude:	N/E	
Neg. Rel. Accom.:	N/E	
Pos. Rel. Accom.:	N/E	
Fused X-Cyl.:	+2.00	
Stereo:	N/E	

Assessment

Moderate compound hyperopic astigmatism and presbyopia.

Plan

We increase GH's spectacle lens prescription to

OD: +2.50 –0.50 × 50/+1.50
OS: +2.25 –0.50 × 155/+1.50

1. The spectacle lens prescription for the right eye preserves the spherical equivalent distance power of the right contact lens (+2.25) and the spherical equivalent near power of the left contact lens (+3.50).
2. Although more plus lens power is accepted at distance on the subjective refraction, we again adopt a conservative approach in increasing distance plus lens power. There is no reason to exceed the plus lens effect of the contact lens prescription when the patient is asymptomatic.
3. Although more cylindrical power is determined on the subjective refraction for the right eye, we adopt a conservative approach toward increasing cylinder power because the cylinder axis has shifted considerably. Considerations in changing cylinder power and axis are discussed in detail in Chapter 5.

4. Despite taking what we thought was a generally conservative approach, DR returns with her glasses complaining that they are "too strong." We reduce her spectacle lens prescription to
   OD: +2.25 –0.50 × 50/+1.50
   OS: +1.75 –0.50 × 155/+1.50

As we see through these case examples, conservative changes are the order of the day when prescribing for patients with hyperopia. Unlike most patients with myopia, patients with hyperopia tend to adopt a certain steady-state tonus of accommodation that is not changed easily, particularly when they are asymptomatic. Symptomatic patients usually accept a small increase in plus lens power. In cases where accommodation or binocular function is compromised, multifocals, prism, or active vision therapy should be considered. These factors are elaborated in Chapter 7, which addresses refractive considerations in binocular vision care.

A final factor, which we have not addressed in this chapter, is spectacle lens design for the patient with hyperopia. It is less of an issue than for patients with appreciable myopia and astigmatism, but the same general guidelines apply. Aspheric lenses typically are used for patients with higher amounts of hyperopia, and a variety of lens materials and indices are available to reduce lens mass and weight. As with any spectacle lens prescription, when the examiner has reason to believe that the patient will be visually sensitive, be cautious about providing new eyewear that significantly changes lens variables such as interpupillary distance, lens material, base curve, pantoscopic angle, or vertex distance.

References

1. Scheiman M, Wick B. *Clinical Management of Binocular Vision.* Philadelphia: Lippincott, 1994:347.
2. Griffin JR, Grisham JD. *Binocular Anomalies*, 3rd ed. Boston: Butterworth–Heinemann, 1995:212.
3. Grisham JD, Simons HD. Refractive error and the reading process: A literature analysis. *J Am Optom Assoc.* 1986;57:44–55.

4. Rosner J, Rosner J. Differences in the perceptual skills development of young myopes and hyperopes. *Am J Optom Physiol Opt.* 1985;62:501–504.

5. Rosenfield M. Refractive status of the eye. In: WJ Benjamin (ed). *Borish's Clinical Refraction.* Philadelphia: Saunders, 1998:9.

6. Hofstetter HW, Griffin JR, Berman MS, Everson RW. *Dictionary of Visual Science and Related Clinical Terms*, 5th ed. Boston: Butterworth–Heinemann, 2000:237.

7. Amos JF. Cycloplegic refraction. In: JD Bartlett, SD Jaanus (eds). *Clinical Ocular Pharmacology*, 4th ed. Boston: Butterworth–Heinemann, 2001:427.

8. Carlson NB, Kurtz D, Heath DA, Hines C. *Clinical Procedures for Ocular Examination*, 2nd ed. Stamford, CT: Appleton and Lange, 1996:131.

9. Miranda MN. Residual accommodation. A comparison between cyclopentolate 1% and a combination of cyclopentolate 1% and tropicamide 1%. *Arch Ophthalmol.* 1972;87:151–171.

10. Blaho KE, Connor CG, Winbery SI. Pharmacology and refraction. In: WJ Benjamin (ed). *Borish's Clinical Refraction.* Philadelphia: Saunders, 1998:376.

11. Birnbaum MH. *Optometric Management of Nearpoint Vision Disorders.* Boston: Butterworth–Heinemann, 1993:62.

12. Manas L. *Visual Analysis Handbook.* Chicago: Professional Press, 1952:57.

13. Editorial: The distance prescription. *J Behav Optom.* 1999;10:2,17.

14. Rosner J, Rosner J. Some observations of the relationship between the visual perceptual skills development of young hyperopes and age of first lens correction. *Clin and Exper Optom.* 1986;69:166–168.

15. Matthews GG. *Neurobiology: Molecules, Cells, and Systems*, 2nd ed. Malden, MA: Blackwell Science, 2001:488–490.

CHAPTER 5

Prescribing for the Patient with Astigmatism

Sir Isaac Newton is credited with being the first scientist to consider astigmatism in detail, although it was not until 1827 that Airy first corrected astigmatism with a cylindrical lens.[1] Uncompensated astigmatism creates a degree of blur that increases with magnitude but varies with the axis of orientation. Given similar amounts of uncompensated astigmatism, blur is relatively greatest when the axis is oblique; least when the axis is with the rule; and in between when the axis is against the rule. This gives rise to predictive guides correlating the amount and orientation of uncorrected astigmatism with uncorrected Snellen acuity values (Table 5-1).

When there is mixed astigmatism, particularly when the spherical equivalent is close to plano, the amount of blur is tempered by the amount of hyperopia, the amount of astigmatism, and the axis of astigmatism. For example, if the subjective refraction yields +0.50 −1.00 × 180 or axis 90, the patient likely sees 20/20 (6/6) without correction. However, if the refraction is +0.50 −1.00 but closer to axis 45 or 135, uncorrected acuity is closer to 20/25 (6/7.5). If the refraction is +1.00 −2.00 × 180 or axis 90, uncorrected acuity is likely to be close to 20/25 (6/7.5) but if the axis is closer to 45 or 135, uncorrected acuity is closer to 20/30 (6/9).

Prescribing for astigmatism often involves a trade-off between maximum comfort and maximum clarity. One school of thought advises prescribing the full cylindrical refraction to every patient and dealing with any maladaptive situations after the fact.[2] We much prefer anticipating how readily the patient will

101

Table 5-1   Expected Relationship of Snellen Acuity to Uncorrected Astigmatism

	Astigmatism		
Snellen Acuity	*Oblique*	*Against the Rule*	*With the Rule*
20/25	0.25	0.50	0.50
20/30	0.75	1.00	1.00
20/40	1.00	1.25	1.50
20/50	1.50	1.75	2.00
20/70	1.75	2.00	2.50
20/100	2.25	2.50	3.00
20/150	2.75	3.00	3.50
20/200	3.50	4.00	4.50

Source: Adapted from Brookman KE. Clinical analysis and management of ametropia. In: KE Brookman (ed). *Refractive Management of Ametropia*. Boston: Butterworth–Heinemann, 1996:5.

handle a prescription change. This minimizes, although it does not realistically eliminate, the need for rechecking what was prescribed when the patient has difficulty adapting to a new prescription. When a recheck of what was prescribed shows the new eyewear to be correct, patients who report having difficulty with their new eyewear should be encouraged to try to adapt to them for a week or two. In most instances, the patient with adaptive difficulty does best in putting away the previous prescription and wearing the new prescription full time.

Patients who are hypercritical and sensitive to very small incremental changes during refraction warrant relatively conservative changes. Patients who are more easygoing and less discriminating when comparing lens changes during the subjective refraction are likely to tolerate larger changes.[3] These points are reflected in the case of patient LB.

Subjective

Case History, Including Signs, Symptoms, and Visual Needs

Patient LB, a 59-year-old retiree, decided to become more serious about his golf game. He brings in a paper bag with a collection of glasses, a sure sign that he is going to be a refractive challenge. We limit the discussion to what he labeled his *old glasses,* in contrast with another pair that he used as his daily (his habitual prescription) and a third pair of glasses that were prescribed for golf but which he was unable to use comfortably. He was dissatisfied because it distorted his judgment of the green, but when he voiced his displeasure, the other doctor insisted that the prescription was correct. Actually, LB was not really pleased with any of his glasses.

Lensometry 1 (old prescription):	OD: $-0.75 -1.25 \times 93 / +1.50$
(FT-28 bifocal):	OS: $-0.75 -1.00 \times 90 / +1.50$
Lensometry 2 (habitual prescription):	OD: $-0.50 -1.50 \times 97 / +1.75$
(FT-28 bifocal):	OS: $-0.50 -1.00 \times 85 / +1.75$
Lensometry 3 (golf):	OD: $-0.25 -1.50 \times 100$
	OS: $-0.25 -1.00 \times 85$

Objective

Ocular Health Assessment

N/E

Clinical Measures

	At 20 ft (6 m)	At 16 in. (40 cm)
VA (habitual	OD: 20/20 (6/6)	20/20 (6/6)
prescription):	OS: 20/20 (6/6)	20/20 (6/6)
Cover Test:	Ortho	Sl exop
N.P.C.:	N/E	
Retinoscopy/	OD: $-0.75 -1.50 \times 100$	
Autorefractor:	OS: $-0.75 -1.00 \times 85$	
Subjective:	OD: $-0.75 -1.25 \times 98$	VA 20/20 (6/6)
	OS: $-0.75 -0.75 \times 76$	VA 20/20 (6/6)
Phoria:	1 exop	4 exop
Base-in vergences:	N/E	N/E
Base-out vergences:	N/E	N/E
Accom. Amplitude:	N/E	
Neg. Rel. Accom.:	N/E	
Pos. Rel. Accom.:	N/E	

Fused X-Cyl.: +2.00 Add, giving 20/20 (6/6) in each eye at 16 in. (40 cm)

Stereo: 20 seconds of arc

Assessment

Compound myopic astigmatism OU with presbyopia OU.

Plan

1. Based on trial framing, we prescribe a new distance bifocal prescription:
   OD: $-0.75 -1.25 \times 95 /+2.00$
   OS: $-0.75 -0.75 \times 80 /+2.00$
2. Based on trial framing (patient lining up a golf ball with a club), we prescribe a single-vision prescription for golf with a 5% amber tint:
   OD: Plano -1.25×95
   OS: Plano -0.75×80

LB's main goal is to obtain a prescription he could use comfortably for golf that would help him "read the green" better. Cylindrical prescriptions may make letters sharper but can have a distorting effect in certain environments, where spatial judgment is paramount. Taking a look at the prescription given to LB by his previous doctor, it appears that he accepted more minus sphere and less cylinder. We are confident that, by reducing the cylindrical component of the prescription at distance as well as lessening the spherocylindrical value of the golf prescription, LB would be pleased.

LB returns to our office with his new prescriptions, stating that the general-purpose bifocal lenses are fine but that he still has trouble judging the green when playing golf. He mentions that his previous doctor had gone through a number of different prescription possibilities before giving up, and it seems like he had to compromise between the lenses that provided best clarity while sacrificing some acuity to minimize spatial distortion. When patients have difficulty with spatial distortion, the best approach includes one or all of three strategies:

1. Reduce the overall cylindrical value, maintaining the same spherical equivalent.
2. Approach equality in the cylindrical power values.
3. Approach symmetry in the cylindrical axis orientation.

In LB's case, we reduced the cylinder by –0.25 diopter in each eye in his unhappy golf prescription, but it proved inadequate. We therefore compromised further and wrote a new prescription based on trial framing that equalized the cylinder power, made the axes symmetrical, and provided a reasonable range of clarity:

OD: –0.25 –0.75 × 90
OS: Plano –0.75 × 90

For visually sensitive patients, the prescriptions we derive may be the best compromise available in clarity versus comfort. The maxim here is that you need not attain perfection to improve on the patient's habitual state. Or, as LB said to us, "I don't expect you to make it perfect. I'm just looking for it be a little bit better."

Adaptation to Cylindrical Changes

Clinical pearl 14 suggests that it is hard to improve on the asymptomatic state. If the patient is happy with his or her lens power and visual acuity is adequate, do not change the prescription.[4] This is particularly true with astigmatism, because changes in cylindrical power exert meridional effects on spatial perception. When meridional image size changes are made, the effect is not just to change size in one meridian but to change the shape of the object as well. Most patients adapt well to these changes if the perceptual shift is offset by an increase in clarity or decrease in asthenopia. When the patient has been happy with the habitual prescription, the perceptual shift induced by changes in cylinder power is more likely to be troublesome.

Small changes in cylinder power, such as 0.25 D or 0.50 D, usually can be tolerated with little difficulty. These changes should be considered strongly when the patient has asthenopic symptoms. Small, uncompensated astigmatic errors can result in significant symptoms because the patient is continually exerting accommodative effort to place the circle of least confusion on the retina.[5] When the change in the amount of cylinder change is larger, more consideration must be given to tempering the prescription. When the change in astigmatic power contemplated for one eye is significantly greater than the fellow eye, binocular aniseikonic effects are created that can be disruptive and trial framing the potential change is warranted. The same holds true for a change in axis orientation, which is of significance when rotated 15° or more on cylinder values above 0.50 D. With higher amounts of astigmatism, smaller degrees of axis change become significant.

Empirical guidelines are useful in deciding how much cylindrical axis shift generally can be tolerated as a function of dioptric cylinder value. Generally speaking, children can tolerate larger cylindrical changes than adults, as they are said to have more cortical plasticity. However, patients of any age can be sensitive to cylindrical changes, as illustrated by patient JV.

Subjective

Case History, Including Signs, Symptoms, and Visual Needs

Patient JV is a 14-year-old high school student, consistently near the top of his class in grades. He is somewhat eccentric and spends most of his free time on the Internet. Ocular history includes a 6-month period of vision therapy for intermittent alternating exotropia. His father reports that JV's eyes have remained straight, and JV is asymptomatic at this time. In fact, he moved up his yearly appointment only because his glasses broke.

Lensometry
OD: −2.25 −1.25 × 31
OS: −2.00 −1.75 × 155

Objective

Ocular Health Assessment
N/E

Clinical Measures

	At 20 ft (6 m)	*At 16 in. (40 cm)*
VA (habitual	OD: 20/25 (6/7.5)	20/25 (6/7.5)
prescription):	OS: 20/25 (6/7.5)	20/25 (6/7.5)
Cover Test:	12 exop	8 exop
N.P.C.:	To the nose	
Retinoscopy/	OD: $-2.50 - 2.00 \times 21$	
Autorefractor:	OS: $-1.75 - 2.25 \times 140$	
Subjective:	OD: $-2.25 - 1.75 \times 22$	VA 20/20 (6/6)
	OS: $-1.75 - 2.25 \times 143$	VA 20/20 (6/6)
Phoria:	12 exop	4 exop
Base-in vergences:	X/12/7	X/22/16
Base-out vergences:	Suppr	X/24/14
Accom. Amplitude:	8 D OD/OS	
Neg. Rel. Accom.:	+1.50	
Pos. Rel. Accom.:	-1.75	
Fused X-Cyl.:	+0.75	
Stereo:	40 seconds of arc	

Assessment

Compound myopic astigmatism OU with mild divergence excess.

Plan

1. We are not going to address JV's binocular status because his fusion, although not perfect, is stable relative to his last visit. Always address the primary reason why the patient came in, which, in JV's case, is simply to replace his glasses. Our instinct was to respect **clinical pearl 14**, which advises against trying to improve on the asymptomatic state and to reissue JV's habitual prescription.
2. What if the temptation is great to resist **clinical pearl 14**? After all, JV did notice the difference between his habitual prescription and his new refraction. So why withhold the increased clarity? We all seem to have a general compulsion to make a slight change in the prescription. Although some may argue with the psychology behind this compulsion, we believe it is based in part on the tendency to justify the need for

the examination when the patient is asymptomatic. Perhaps, we are insecure that the patient might think, "I knew things hadn't changed, so why did they have to examine my vision if they were just going to give me the same prescription?" In time, we overcome this insecurity and do what is in the patient's best interests without overthinking the situation.

Regrettably, in this case, we do not follow our instincts to leave well enough alone and decide to prescribe the subjective findings. After all, it represents an increase of only in 0.50 D cylinder in both eyes and an axis shift of 9° in the right eye and 12° in the left. We figure that a 14 year old who spends most of his time indoors riveted to the computer when not in class should have no difficulty adapting to this change. We were wrong. When JV comes in for his new glasses, he immediately notices some slanting of straight edges. He is a more sensitive and critical observer than we give him credit for being. Although we tell him that he will adjust to his new prescription by wearing it steadily for a week or two, he comes back in three days saying that he is getting headaches and would rather have his old glasses. We redid his lenses to match his previous prescription, and JV was happier.

Subjective

Case History, Including Signs, Symptoms, and Visual Needs

MF is a 54-year-old man who lists his occupation as medical marketing and education. He wears his contact lenses often; these are CSI lenses with a spherical power of –2.00 OD and –1.25 OS. He occasionally leaves out the left lens to create a monovision effect, using the right eye for distance and the left eye for near. He is asymptomatic and has decided to come to the office for examination to try out his company's new vision plan. Since the plan offers coverage for either glasses or contact lenses in any given year, his thought is to obtain prescription sunglasses.

Lensometry
OD: –1.75 –0.75 × 180
OS: –0.75 –1.00 × 10

Objective

Ocular Health Assessment

N/E

Clinical Measures

		At 20 ft (6 m)	*At 16 in. (40 cm)*
VA (habitual	OD:	20/20 (6/6)	20/20 (6/6) sc
prescription):	OS:	20/20 (6/6)	20/25 (6/7.5) sc
Cover Test:		Ortho	Sl exop
N.P.C.:		To the nose (sc)	
Keratometry:	OD:	43.50/44.75 × 180	
	OS:	43.75/45.00 × 10	
Retinoscopy/	OD:	–1.50 –1.00 × 177	
Autorefractor:	OS:	–0.75 –0.75 × 5	
Subjective:	OD:	–1.50 –1.00 × 177	VA 20/20 (6/6)
	OS:	–0.75 –0.75 × 5	VA 20/20 (6/6)
Phoria:		1 exop	5 exop
Base-in vergences:		N/E	N/E
Base-out vergences:		N/E	N/E
Accom. Amplitude:		N/E	
Neg. Rel. Accom.:		N/E	
Pos. Rel. Accom.:		N/E	
Fused X-Cyl.:		+2.00	
Stereo:		N/E	

Assessment

Compound myopic astigmatism OU with low anisometropia and presbyopia.

Plan

1. We prescribe the distance subjective as a prescription sun lens in single-vision form.
2. We do not suggest that the patient try a multifocal for his sun lens, as he is happy removing his distance prescription for reading. This gives him a spherical equivalent add of 2 diopters with the right eye.

You may wonder why, in this case, we are giving patient MF a sun lens prescription that differs from his habitual lens prescription. This seems to violate **clinical pearl 14**, which suggests that we not try to improve on the asymptomatic state. True enough; and we would not quibble with someone who decides to issue the same prescription in the sun lens as MF has in his habitual prescription, with which he is happy. We take into account that, if we make a slight change in cylindrical value and the patient does not appear to be too discerning or visually sensitive during the subjective, then the power change should be accepted readily. We predict that patient MF should have no difficulty switching back and forth between the two prescriptions because they are very similar. However, you may want to plant the seed with MF that, if he feels more comfortable and appreciates better clarity with his sunglasses prescription, he should change his nonsunglasses prescription to match it.

Spatial Distortion and Trial Framing

We mentioned earlier several approaches to minimizing spatial distortion. When the amount of cylinder in the tentative prescription is greater than a 0.50 D change from the habitual prescription, recheck to determine if the patient can see just as well with less cylinder by adjusting the sphere value. **Clinical pearl 10** is a reminder that, in maintaining the spherical equivalent, you always need to adjust the value of the sphere when you change the power of the cylinder. For example, if the patient's habitual prescription is –0.50 –1.25 × 180 OU and your refraction is –0.50 –2.25 × 180, doublecheck to see if the patient can see just as well with –0.75 –1.75 × 180.

The second approach to minimizing spatial distortion is to approach equality in the cylindrical power values. This is particularly important when the cylindrical axes are oblique. For example, if the habitual prescription is

OD: –1.25 –0.50 × 145
OS: –1.25 –0.50 × 35

and the refraction is

OD: −0.75 −1.50 × 145
OS: −1.25 −0.75 × 35

consider prescribing

OD: −1.00 −1.00 × 145
OS: −1.25 −0.75 × 35

With each of these strategies, trial framing is important when you suspect that the patient is sensitive to small changes. In the preceding example, there's a distinct possibility that **clinical pearl 15** is operative. When first glancing at the difference in the habitual prescription and the refraction, we may think that the previous doctor simply failed to determine the full cylindrical power. But the patient's last doctor may be wiser than initially realized and purposely undercorrected the cylinder power. A good clue to this is to ask the patient if he or she recalls having difficulty getting adjusted to previous glasses. The patient may then volunteer that at first the previous glasses made things look strange, so the doctor rewrote the prescription.

When the current refraction shows a cylinder axis significantly different from the habitual prescription and the cylindrical power is less than 1 diopter, consider eliminating the cylinder and prescribing the spherical equivalent. For example, if the habitual prescription is

OD: −6.00 −0.50 × 100
OS: −6.25 −0.50 × 70

and the refraction is

OD: −6.00 −0.50 × 165
OS: −6.25 −0.50 × 175

consider prescribing

OD: −6.25 sphere
OS: −6.50 sphere

This situation is encountered most commonly when a patient wears rigid gas-permeable (RGP) contact lenses all day and uses glasses only to read or watch television briefly before bedtime, although it may occur with any patient.

The third strategy to minimize spatial distortion is to modify the cylindrical axes to make them less oblique or more symmetrical. Minimizing the change toward oblique axes orientation helps reduce spatial distortion. For example, if the habitual prescription is OU −4.25 −1.50 × 180 and the refraction is

OD: −4.00 −1.50 × 150
OS: −4.00 −1.50 × 30

consider prescribing

OD: −4.25 −1.50 × 165
OS: −4.25 −1.50 × 15

Minimizing the change toward asymmetric axes is accomplished in the following example. If the habitual prescription is OU −4.25 −1.50 × 180 and the refraction is

OD: −4.25 −1.50 × 180
OS: −4.25 −1.50 × 160

consider prescribing

OD: −4.25 −1.50 × 180
OS: −4.25 −1.50 × 170

Although we tend to think of problems with spatial distortion induced by higher cylindrical powers, relatively low cylindrical power can be problematic as well, particularly when the patient has not previously worn glasses. Such was the case with patient RR.

Subjective

Case History, Including Signs, Symptoms, and Visual Needs

Patient RR, a 42-year-old sales representative, started to notice some difficulty in focusing on small print. We examined him last year, and although he was asymptomatic at the time, we advised him that he was on the cusp of presbyopia and likely would notice difficulty with focusing at near during the next year. He still takes the same medications, which are Lipitor to control his cholesterol, Glucotrol to control his blood sugar, vitamin B-12, and folic acid. His most recent medical examination, 3 months ago, showed his cholesterol and blood sugar levels to be normal.

Objective

Ocular Health Assessment

External examination and vitreoretinal structures were normal. There were no ocular signs of systemic disease.

Clinical Measures

		At 20 ft (6 m)	*At 16 in. (40 cm)*
VA (uncorrected):	OD:	20/25 (6/7.5)	20/30 (6/9)
	OS:	20/25 (6/7.5)	20/25 (6/7.5)
Cover Test:		Ortho	Sl exop
N.P.C.:		N/E	
Retinoscopy/	OD:	+0.75 –0.50 × 135	
Autorefractor:	OS:	+1.00 –1.00 × 60	
Subjective:	OD:	+0.50 –0.50 × 135	VA 20/20
	OS:	+0.50 –1.00 × 60	VA 20/20
Phoria:		N/E	N/E
Base-in vergences:		N/E	N/E
Base-out vergences:		N/E	N/E
Accom. Amplitude:		5 D	
Neg. Rel. Accom.:		N/E	
Pos. Rel. Accom.:		N/E	
Fused X-Cyl.:		+1.50 through distance prescription	
Stereo:		40 seconds of arc	

Assessment

Compound hyperopic astigmatism OD with mixed astigmatism OS.

Plan

1. Patient RR has no complaint about his distance vision. We want to give him a prescription that not only increases clarity for small print but would not be unnecessarily strong or disorienting when he looks up. He does not want to feel the need to remove his glasses every time he speaks to a client or gets up from his desk briefly. Since the cylinder axes are oblique and RR has not previously worn glasses, the probability is that he would have been symptomatic with the full cylinder prescribed. Based on trial framing, we arrive at the following prescription, which improves near clarity yet does not bother RR when he looks up or walks around:
   OD: +1.00 –0.50 × 135
   OS: +1.00 –0.50 × 60

2. Patient RR returns to our office 1 month after receiving his eyewear, stating that he could not wear his prescription at the computer. He felt bad but really did try hard to adjust to the prescription. Nevertheless, in his words, "they made the screen look like a parallelogram." In fact, someone gave him over-the-counter glasses, which were the weakest strength, and everything seemed more comfortable. He brought them in for us to check the power, and they were +0.75 sph OU.

3. We remade the prescription as +0.75 sph OU. Even though we thought we were being conservative by prescribing cylinder in equal amounts for both eyes and trial framing did not elicit a feeling of spatial distortion, there are times when sensitive patients do not experience symptoms until they use their first prescriptive lenses in the everyday work environment.

4. What other options are there in this case? We could have remade the lenses with less cylinder, reducing them to 0.25 in each eye. We also might have tried to prescribe the cylinder axes with less obliquity, perhaps arbitrarily changing each cylinder by 15° toward axis 90. This would change the

right axis from 135 to 120 and the left axis from 60 to 75. Certainly both variables could be changed at once, resulting in a new prescription for near of

OD: +1.00 –0.25 × 120
OS: +1.00 –0.25 × 75

Those favoring such an approach might suggest that it is important for the patient to feel that he or she has a primary pair of glasses that account for the astigmatism, rather than relying on over-the-counter glasses. In this case, we feel comfortable prescribing what the patient told us he is comfortable with. The final decision is going to be a judgment call.

A similarly challenging case is the new patient who comes to the office principally because he lost his glasses, and you have no previous prescription with which to compare the refraction. This is the case with patient MF.

Subjective

Case History, Including Signs, Symptoms, and Visual Needs

Patient MF is a 47-year-old consultant who recently lost his glasses. He had been using them primarily for driving and felt fine reading and using the computer without them. His general health is fine, and he tends to avoid going to the eye doctor because he always dreaded getting new glasses. But his wife and daughter mentioned that they had a very pleasant experience in our office, and losing his glasses left him with less of an excuse to delay having his eyes examined. He felt okay with his previous glasses but noticed that he seemed to have to work at refocusing his eyes whenever he took his glasses off, so he tried to use them as little as possible. In MF's words, he felt like his glasses gave him "a visual hangover."

Lensometry

Glasses were lost. His last exam was 5 years ago, but that doctor retired and they were unable to locate his file in the office that took over the previous doctor's records.

Objective

Ocular Health Assessment

N/E

Clinical Measures

		At 20 ft (6 m)	At 16 in. (40 cm)
VA (habitual	OD:	20/50 (6/15)	20/25 (6/7.5)
prescription):	OS:	20/50 (6/15)	20/25 (6/7.5)
Cover Test:		Sl exop	Sl exop
N.P.C.:		N/E	
Retinoscopy/	OD:	−1.50 −0.75 × 117	
Autorefractor:	OS:	−1.50 −1.50 × 73	
Subjective:	OD:	−1.25 −0.75 × 115	VA 20/20 (6/6)
	OS:	−1.25 −1.50 × 75	VA 20/20 (6/6)
Phoria:		Ortho	3 exop
Base-in vergences:		N/E	N/E
Base-out vergences:		N/E	N/E
Accom. Amplitude:		4 D OD/OS	
Neg. Rel. Accom.:		+2.50	
Pos. Rel. Accom.:		−1.00	
Fused X-Cyl.:		+1.25	
Stereo:		N/E	

Assessment

Compound myopic astigmatism OU and early presbyopia.

Plan

1. One could make a strong argument for prescribing the subjective refraction and assume that it is close to his habitual prescription. By the same token, MF uses his prescription principally for driving, so we should be careful about spatial perception. Since his glasses are not worn full ime, adaptation is more challenging. Recall as well that he notes effort in refocusing his eyes whenever he takes off his glasses and therefore tries to use them as little as possible. This usually is due to cylindrical effects, accommodative inertia, or a combination of both factors.

2. We modify MF's prescription slightly so that we provide good clarity but minimize factors that would result in his feeling of "a visual hangover" when he removes the glasses. Specifically, we reduce the minus sphere and minimize the cylindrical asymmetry in power and axes to arrive at the following prescription:
OD: −1.00 −0.75 × 105
OS: −1.25 −1.00 × 75

It is fine to alter a prescription intentionally to find the most comfortable vision rather than the sharpest. However, if the compromise between comfort and clarity results in something less than 20/20 (6/6) acuity, be sure to explain to the patient what you are doing and why and be sure to note in your record the acuity is through the lens that you prescribe. We encounter an extreme case of tempering cylindrical power with patient SE.

Subjective

Case History, Including Signs, Symptoms, and Visual Needs
Patient SE, a 45-year-old computer technician, was injured a number of years ago while serving in the military. He describes his injury as a tear of the iris, which was repaired, but notes that the vision in his right eye has been poorer than the left eye ever since. SE is wearing his previous pair of glasses, with which he is comfortable. He went to a new optometrist last year because of eye care coverage through work but is dissatisfied. Actually, he expresses his dissatisfaction graphically: Reportedly, when Doctor Plan dispensed the new glasses to SE, he advised him that he would "see like a hawk." As SE expresses, he feels like a hawk all right—a cross-eyed hawk because he is seeing double. When he returned to complain about his glasses, the doctor checked them and told SE that they were correct and that he would just have to get used to them. The lensometry findings for the two prescriptions are as follows.
Habitual prescription,

OD: −2.50 −0.75 × 66/+1.25
OS: −2.50 −0.25 × 130/+1.25

Newer prescription,

OD: −1.25 −2.00 × 115/+1.25
OS: −2.75 sphere/+1.25

Objective

Ocular Health Assessment

The iris structures in both eyes look perfectly normal despite the patient's comment that the iris of the right eye had been injured. However, there were numerous striae of the right cornea. All other eye health findings were normal.

Clinical Measures

	At 20 ft (6 m)	At 16 in. (40 cm)
VA (habitual prescription):	OD: 20/40 (6/12)	20/40 (6/12)
	OS: 20/20 (6/6)	20/20 (6/6)
Cover Test:	Ortho	Sl exop
N.P.C.:	N/E	
Retinoscopy/ Autorefractor:	OD: −0.25 −4.00 × 105 (keratometry OD: 40.00/43.73 × 112 with mires moderately distorted)	
	OS: −2.50 −0.50 × 131	
Subjective:	OD: −0.75 −2.50 × 70	VA 20/25 (6/7.5)
	OS: −2.50 −0.50 × 130	VA 20/20 (6/6)
Phoria:	Diplopia, unable to neutralize with prism. Central suppression OD through habitual prescription.	
Base-in vergences:	None	None
Base-out vergences:	None	None
Accom. Amplitude:	N/E	
Neg. Rel. Accom.:	N/E	
Pos. Rel. Accom.:	N/E	
Fused X-Cyl.:	+1.50 through habitual distance prescription	
Stereo:	N/E	

Assessment

Acquired, long-standing anisometropic astigmatism due to corneal injury, with early presbyopia.

Plan

1. We decide to reissue SE's habitual prescription.
2. On refraction, with the lens providing best acuity for the right eye in place, SE remarks that he sees sharply. But when both eyes are open, he sees two eye charts. The prescription previously given him induced sufficient blur to allow SE to suppress centrally. SE had long-adapted to a comfortable balance between the sharpest acuity possible and the most comfortable binocular (or at least bi-ocular) vision.
3. We realize that, in some instances, an optometrist feels compelled to make some change in prescription. Some small changes might be made based on the subjective findings relative to the habitual prescription, but be cautious about rocking the boat when a patient is pleased with the habitual prescription and displeased with the most recent prescription.

Patient SE represents a dramatic example of trading off best cylindrical acuity for best cylindrical comfort. Bear in mind that, in much subtler cases, patients express a preference for changes that you would not think likely to bother them. Some patients feel that lenses prescribed for them are too strong, even when they involve very low cylindrical values. It might be the difference between a patient accepting a prescription of plano –0.25 but feeling that plano –0.50, which is what he or she accepted behind the phoropter, is too strong. You cannot always identify which patients fall into this category beforehand, but it would be unfair to label all such nonadapters as neurotic. An entire school of thought says that some cylindrical shifts occur as signs of visual problems rather than as causes of a visual problem requiring compensation with prescriptions. This is particularly true with low values of against-the-rule astigmatism.[6] The point is that even low cylindrical prescriptive changes can plague sensitive patients who present for routine examination with no complaint of visual change.

We take this opportunity to elaborate on the inclination of some examiners to change a patient's prescription for the sake of change. In a case where the patient is convinced that something has changed with the prescription but the examiner finds no significant change, the patient may needlessly worry if the examiner advises that nothing has changed. Particularly with astigmatism, the opportunity presents itself to change 0.25 D or a couple of degrees and legitimately tell the patient that there has been a slight change in the prescription. The practitioner may elect to tell the patient that the change is mild and that whether or not to change the prescription is something the patient can decide. It puts the patient's mind at ease to know that there is a slight change in the prescription and nothing major is wrong. Pushing the asymptomatic patient toward a change in prescription is an ethical issue and beyond the scope of this discussion.[7]

When the patient comes in with glasses misaligned, badly scratched, or giving some other indication during refraction that this patient is not particularly visually sensitive, do not worry as much about adjusting the cylinder power or axis. But, for the patient who wonders whether the hairline scratch in the lower right corner of his lens warrants replacement, be particularly conservative about changing cylinder power or axis. With visually sensitive patients it is equally important to anticipate adaptive problems stemming from a change in the habitual eyewear related to lens material, base curve, frame size and shape, relative position of optical centers, and pantoscopic angle. We elaborate on these factors in the next section.

The Visually Sensitive Patient

A number of clues indicate to the examiner that the patient is sensitive to small visual changes. There may be a notation to this effect in the record if the patient has been evaluated previously in that office or clinic. When the patient relates that he or she has had numerous glasses, none of which has been "right," this is another clue. If you are examining the patient for the first time, the most obvious sign of visual sensitivity is the ability to discriminate between very small variations in spherocylinder power or cylinder axis.

As discussed earlier in this chapter, individual sensitivity to cylindrical effects varies considerably, as does perception of spatial distortion with changes in lens power or form. Patients who have difficulty with cylindrical changes report that surfaces appear slanted or tilted. Although you might think that trial framing the patient would elicit these symptoms, it often does not. Even though trial framing is advisable, bear in mind that the trial lenses are small and round and have flat base curves. All this tends to minimize spatial distortion. The best way to solve adaptive problems is to try to prevent them. Therefore, when dealing with a patient you suspect of being visually sensitive, use empirical guidelines in anticipating difficulties associated with a change in lens prescription or material. We list such guidelines in Table 5-2, and each warrants some consideration.

1. *Change in cylinder axis or power too large.* Suggested guidelines are given in Table 5-3 regarding conservative changes in cylinder power and axis.
2. *Change in lens material or index of refraction.* Although lens material with higher indices of refraction are popular when trying to minimize lens weight or thickness, visually sensitive patients should be advised that they may perceive some change from what they were used to but this resolves within

Table 5-2   Checklist for Problems in Prescription Adaptation

___ Change in cylinder axis or power too large

___ Change in lens material or index of refraction

___ Change in base curve or asphericity

___ Change in frame shape or size

___ Position of optical centers

___ Change in pantoscopic angle

___ Change in monocular or binocular PD

___ Excyclotorsion effect at near

Table 5-3   Suggested Guidelines for Maximum Axis Change

Change in Cylinder Value	Suggested Change in Degrees
0.25–0.50	Unlimited
0.75–1.25	≤45
1.50–2.00	≤30
>–2.00	≤10

Example:
Habitual prescription: –1.00 –0.50 × 90
Refraction: –1.00 –1.25 × 30
New prescription: –1.00 –1.25 × 60

a few days. A change to a higher index material necessitates a flatter base curve and decreased center thickness, resulting in altered shape magnification.[8]

3. *Change in base curve or asphericity.* When we know the patient is visually sensitive, have the laboratory match the habitual base curves as closely as possible. When previous information tells you the patient is visually sensitive, such has having had to remake prescriptions in the past, or when problem solving, take note of the base curve in the right lens compared to the left. If the patient is more comfortable with previous eyewear and the base curves of the lenses are asymmetrical, preserve the asymmetry. If previous comfortable eyewear had front surface cylinder, request front surface cylinder on the new lenses as well. Aspheric surfaces often are used to enhance lens appearance and optics, but bear in mind that the visually sensitive patient may have trouble adjusting to any change and is less concerned with being offered the latest advances in ophthalmic optics.

4. *Change in monocular or binocular interpupillary distance (PD).* You may measure an anatomical PD that is different from the mechanical PD obtained during lensometry. When the patient is visually sensitive, particularly in higher powers, be conservative about prescribing monocular or binocular PDs that differ from the patient's habitual prescription.

5. *Position of optical centers.* Take note of the monocular position of the optical center in the frame. When the power is high, it is helpful to dot the location of the center of the pupil in the frame with a felt-tipped marker as a reference for the laboratory.

6. *Change frame shape or size.* It is well recognized that frames with angles rather than round shapes tend to induce relatively more distortion, and that small eye sizes (and therefore smaller lenses) tend to minimize lens aberrations, particularly in higher powers. However, the visually sensitive patient again is called on to make an adaptation if switching to a frame of considerably different shape or size. Encourage the patient to make moderate rather than radical changes in lens size or shape. For example, going with smaller eye sizes generally results in less spatial distortion. However, when visually sensitive, the patient may be bothered by an increased awareness of the border of the frame or lens. The opposite may occur for a patient with a narrow PD, who switches to a rimless frame with a drill mount and is now distracted by the position of the inner mount assembly describing it as "something's just not right with these new glasses."

7. *Change in pantoscopic angle.* A change in pantoscopic angle alters the cylindrical effects of the lenses. As pantoscopic angle increases, lens distortion is likely to increase. However, we return to the observation that the sensitive patient who has adapted to the habitual state will find any change challenging, even if it theoretically should improve the optical image. Therefore, if the patient typically has a greater than average degree of pantoscopic tilt, try to reproduce it in the new eyewear. As a general rule, keeping the frame adjusted so that the lenses are as close to the eyes as possible minimizes spatial distortion.

8. *Excylotorsion effect at near.* When a patient with astigmatism finds distance adequate in a new prescription but has difficulty with near vision that is unrelated to the spherical equivalent lens power, suspect excyclotorsion as the culprit. When the near complaints cannot be explained through

abnormal binocular findings, check the refraction at near to see if the patient takes a different spherocylinder power for maximum acuity and comfort. This usually is not a factor unless the patient has a high amount of cylinder in one or both eyes.

Any of these factors may occur individually or collectively, and they always are magnified when occurring with visually sensitive patients, as was the case with patient MB.

Subjective

Case History, Including Signs, Symptoms, and Visual Needs
MB is a 39-year-old homemaker who studied interior design. She served in the military, is very exacting, and has an eye for detail. From an optometrist's point of view, she may be a bit too sensitive to visual detail. She scheduled an appointment to replace an RGP contact lens that recently was lost, and said that we came highly recommended to her from a friend. MB is pleased with her current glasses and RGP contact lenses, and her personal and family medical and ocular histories are unremarkable. Based on the history and findings, we decide to prescribe the same spectacle lens power, and MB has the prescription filled elsewhere. She returns the day after receiving her glasses, complaining that, when she put them on, there was a sensation that her eyes were pulling inward.

Lensometry
OD: −4.50 −0.50 × 80
OS: −4.00 −1.00 × 80

Objective

Ocular Health Assessment
All eye health findings are normal.

Clinical Measures

	At 20 ft (6 m)	*At 16 in. (40 cm)*
VA (habitual	OD: 20/20 (6/6)	20/20 (6/6)
prescription):	OS: 20/20 (6/6)	20/20 (6/6)
Cover Test:	Ortho	Sl exop
N.P.C.:	N/E	
Retinoscopy/	OD: −4.50 −0.50 × 85	
Autorefractor:	OS: −4.25 −1.00 × 78	
Subjective:	OD: −4.50 −0.50 × 80	VA 20/20 (6/6)
	OS: −4.00 −1.00 × 80	VA 20/20 (6/6)
Phoria:	N/E	N/E
Base-in vergences:	N/E	N/E
Base-out vergences:	N/E	N/E
Accom. Amplitude:	6 D	
Neg. Rel. Accom.:	N/E	
Pos. Rel. Accom.:	N/E	
Fused X-Cyl.:	+0.75 through habitual distance prescription	
Stereo:	N/E	

Assessment

Compound myopic astigmatism OU.

Plan

When MB describes the sensation of her eyes "pulling inward" with the new prescription, our assumption is that the PD is off and she was getting a prismatic effect that results in a convergence effect. But the PD on the new prescription measures 60, and the monocular PDs are symmetrical at 30 mm OD and OS, which is equivalent to her anatomical PD. She therefore has no prescribed or induced lateral prism. We looked at the optical centers between the two sets of eyewear, and they were quite comparable. We then checked the base curves and found the following:

Base curves of habitual prescription: +4.25 with front surface cylinder OU.

Base curves of new prescription: +4.25 with rear surface cylinder OU.

We explain to MB in lay terms how the change in base curve might affect her sensation and perception . She asks me why the source that filled her prescription did not take that into consideration. We related that most people are not sensitive enough to make it practical or cost efficient to check every possible variable before filling every prescription. However, now that we are aware of her sensitivity, in the future we or the firm that fills her prescription will take this into account.

MB admits that she's the first one to walk into a house and notice that a painting is hung crooked. She tells her friends how to rearrange their furniture. She is highly visual and, thinking about it, knows that she is visually hypersensitive. But what do you say to a patient who remarks, "I've been wearing glasses all my life and have never had a problem with new glasses like this before?" We tell the patient to consider the analogy to allergies. It is possible to not have a history of allergies, then to develop a hypersensitivity some time in adulthood. Similarly, the visual system becomes less "plastic" or adaptable in adulthood, and a patient who had more visual flexibility earlier in life can become more sensitive to changes in lens parameters.

We tell MB to put away her other glasses, not wear her contact lenses, and either live in these glasses for two days or have them remade. MB decides to have the lenses remade with front surface cylinder and is happier.

Meridional Amblyopia

Uncompensated astigmatism can serve as a source of abnormal visual experience during a sensitive period of development in young children, thereby resulting in amblyopia.[9] The continued presence of 1.5 or more diopters of astigmatism in 1 year olds that is left uncorrected has been identified as a significant predictor of subsequent amblyopia.[10] Refractive amblyopia due to uncompensated astigmatism can occur either unilaterally due to anisometropic astigmatism or bilaterally due to high uncompensated astigmatism in both eyes.[11] The general tendency is to prescribe more aggressively and more fully for astigmatism in young children to minimize the likelihood of meridional amblyopia (refractive amblyopia caused by uncorrected astigmatism). We follow the guidelines offered by Ciner, indicating full compensation of astigmatism exceeding 1.25 diopters when it is consistent and the child is over 2 years of age.[12] Once identified as having meridional amblyopia, children who are prescribed lenses should be monitored at least once every 6 months initially and no less frequently than yearly thereafter, at least until age 12.[13] Although astigmatism tends to change less dramatically than spherical ametropia in children, this is not always the case, as demonstrated by patient KM.

Subjective

Case History, Including Signs, Symptoms, and Visual Needs

KM is a 5 year old whose mother brought her in for examination because her older sister has high myopia. She passed the vision screening in the pediatrician's office, which is not given until age 5. KM has no visual complaints and her parents have noticed nothing unusual, such as squinting. Her developmental history and motor milestones are normal.

Objective

Ocular Health Assessment

Internal and external eye structures are healthy and normal in appearance. Her optic nerve disks are ovoid, as commonly seen in children with moderate to high amounts of against-the-rule cylinder.

Clinical Measures

	At 20 ft (6 m)	At 16 in. (40 cm)
VA (sc):	OD: 20/40 (6/12)	20/40 (6/12)
	OS: 20/40 (6/12)	20/40 (6/12)
Cover Test:	Ortho	Sl exop
N.P.C.:	To the nose	

	At 20 ft (6 m)	*At 16 in. (40 cm)*
Retinoscopy/	OD: +1.00 −2.50 × 100	
Autorefractor:	OS: +0.50 −2.25 × 80	
Subjective:	OD: +1.00 −2.50 × 100	VA 20/30 (6/9)
	OS: +0.50 −2.25 × 80	VA 20/30 (6/9)
Phoria:	Ortho	4 exop
Base-in vergences:	N/E	N/E
Base-out vergences:	N/E	N/E
Accom. Amplitude:	>10 D OD/OS	
Neg. Rel. Accom.:	N/E	
Pos. Rel. Accom.:	N/E	
Fused X-Cyl.:	+0.75	
Stereo:	40 seconds of arc	

Assessment

Mixed astigmatism with mild bilateral refractive (meridional) amblyopia.

Plan

1. We prescribe KM's subjective refraction for full-time wear. Obtaining 20/30 (6/9) with a 5 year old might be a judgment call, because many 5 year olds typically do not respond to Snellen acuity letters smaller than 20/30 (6/9) when tested at a distance. KM struggles to read 20/40 (6/12) uncorrected and with the prescription lenses reads a crisp 20/30 (6/9) but is hesitant to read the 20/25 (6/7.5) line.

2. We keep KM's prescription the same until age 8, at which time her refraction has increased to:
   OD: −1.00 −2.75 × 87, providing 20/25 (6/7.5) acuity
   OS: −1.50 −2.50 × 87, providing 20/25 (6/7.5) acuity
   Based on trial lens responses, we decided to undercorrect the sphere and prescribe the following:
   OD: −0.50 −2.75 × 87
   OS: −0.50 −2.50 × 87

3. By age 10, KM's retinoscopy has changed to
   OD: −1.25 −3.50 × 90
   OS: −0.75 −3.25 × 88

Her subjective at that time is
OD: $-0.75 -2.75 \times 88$ (20/25)
OS: $-0.50 -2.50 \times 88$ (20/25)

4. At age 11, retinoscopy reveals
OD: $-1.00 -3.75 \times 94$ (20/25)
OS: $-1.00 -4.75 \times 90$ (20/25)
Keratometry:
OD: 41.75/44.25 × 101
OS: 41.75/44.50 × 89
Based on trial framing, we change her prescription to -0.75 -3.25×90, yielding 20/25 (6/7.5) acuity OU.

5. Although we do not do corneal topography to document the nature of corneal changes over time, it is entirely possible that KM is a young keratoconic patient. This would not have influenced how we prescribed for her, however, as long as clear and comfortable acuity could be obtained with glasses. Another possibility is that we began prescribing for KM at too young an age and interfered with the emmetropization process. We think this unlikely, although we could have withheld the prescription at age 5 and simply followed KM every 6 months to make sure her best corrected acuity was not decreasing.

6. Another possibility is that KM experiences some visual stress due to being an early and avid reader. Her older sister is highly myopic and her mother is concerned about KM's rate of myopic progression. There is room to consider prescribing a multifocal prescription or vision therapy in KM's case if we assume that some portion of the astigmatism is adaptive.

Adaptive Astigmatism

A school of thought, formalized by Birnbaum, views low-power, against-the-rule cylindrical refractive findings as adaptive.[14] A sign of this is when the cylinder axis is against the rule and not matched by what a simplified version of Javal's rule predicts. As suggested by Grosvenor, Quintero, and Perrigin, the simplified

Javal's rule predicts that the keratometric cylinder can be combined with –0.50 × 90 to predict the refractive astigmatic power.[15]

As an example, assume that the patient's keratometer reading shows –0.50 × 180. Using the simplified Javal's rule we add –0.50 × 90 to that amount, and the cylindrical values cancel. This would predict that the patient's refraction would be spherical. If the patient refracts with an against-the-rule cylinder, it should be prescribed with caution. We suggest being conservative with a low, adaptive against-the-rule cylinder, because if it indeed is a sign of visual stress, prescribing the cylinder will not solve the visual problem (Table 5-4). Consider reducing or eliminating the cylinder power and adjust the sphere accordingly. Recognizing the presence of accommodative dysfunction or other near-point disorders can help make this decision, as was the case with patient DW.

Subjective

Case History, Including Signs, Symptoms, and Visual Needs
DW is a 23-year-old law student who complains of distance blur. She first noticed the blur last year when looking across the room after studying for sustained periods of time. Gradually, the blur became constant, and she now feels insecure driving at night.

Her general health is good, and she had a full physical exam last month. Although there is a history of diabetes in the family, her blood sugar is normal.

Table 5-4 Guidelines for Prescribing Cylinder

---

1. Prescribe full cylinder if it has been accepted by the patient before.
2. Prescribe full cylinder for a child with refractive amblyopia.
3. Rx the maximum sphere and minimum cylinder for best acuity and comfort.
4. Temper cylindrical changes in axis based on guidelines in Table 5-3.
5. Be wary of spatial distortion with asymmetric oblique cylinders (e.g., X135/X45).
6. Be conservative about astigmatism that appears to be adaptive.

Objective

Ocular Health Assessment

Internal and external eye structures are healthy and normal in appearance.

Clinical Measures

		At 20 ft (6 m)	At 16 in. (40 cm)
VA (sc):	OD:	20/40 (6/12)	20/20 (6/6)
	OS:	20/40 (6/12)	20/20 (6/6)
Cover Test:		Ortho	Sl esop
N.P.C.:		To the nose	
Retinoscopy/	OD:	–0.50 –0.75 × 85	
Autorefractor:	OS:	–0.50 –0.75 × 95	
Subjective:	OD:	–0.50 –0.50 × 90	VA 20/20 (6/6)
	OS:	–0.50 –0.50 × 90	VA 20/20 (6/6)
Phoria:		1 esop	4 esop
Base-in vergences:		4/7/4	8/12/10
Base-out vergences:		X/20/14	X/24/18
Accom. Amplitude:		10 D OD/OS	
Neg. Rel. Accom.:		+1.50	
Pos. Rel. Accom.:		–2.00	
Fused X-Cyl.:		–0.25	
Stereo:		20 seconds of arc	

Assessment

Compound myopic astigmatism OU, likely pseudomyopia secondary to accommodative and convergence excess.

Plan

1. Based on trial frame responses, we give DW a single-vision prescription for –0.50 OU for use at distance, simply omitting the refractive cylinder. When we compare clarity and comfort with –0.75, the –0.50 was preferred.
2. The data do not strongly support prescribing a multifocal; and when we mention this as a possibility to DW, she indicates she does not want to use a multifocal lens.

3. We discuss the option of vision therapy with DW, and she is interested in considering this option when her school demands lighten.

Cases have been reported in the literature of low amounts of against-the-rule astigmatism induced by near-point stress lessening when the patient receives a near-point lens or vision therapy. Although it is uncertain that DW would undertake either option, prescribing the cylinder when it could just as easily be omitted would likely embed the cylinder, ignore the source of the refractive shift, and encourage more myopic progression. This subject is discussed in more detail in Chapter 3.

The Complex Patient with Adaptive Difficulties

At various points during a career, practitioners will encounter patients who have complex personal histories. In some instances, the patient has a history of periodic visual disturbances, is afflicted with known or suspected disease processes, and is taking numerous medications. When the patient has difficulty with a lens prescription, the tendency is to dismiss or minimize the significance of the lens prescription as the source of the problem and attribute it to the patient's nature or perhaps to the cyclical side effects of disease or medication.

However, when a change has been made in the astigmatic power of the patient's lenses, and the patient claims to be more comfortable with previous eyewear (having less astigmatic correction), consider the possibility that the symptoms are due to the refractive change. Such is the case with patient JD.

Subjective

Case History, Including Signs, Symptoms, and Visual Needs
JD is a 59-year-old payroll clerk, first seen in the office 7 years ago. At that time, she was taking Lotensin to control hypertension and Lorazepam for anxiety. She reported that, when her blood pressure was out of control, her vision was noticeably affected. Her anxiety resulted in periodic panic attacks while driving. JD would have to

pull over to the side of the road because, as she described it, she could see but she could not focus properly. At the time of her first examination in the office, JD's prescription was –1.25 –0.50 × 180 OD and –1.25 –0.50 × 150 OS, providing 20/20 (6/6) with each eye at distance. She had transition lenses, which helped with her sensitivity to light not only outdoors but indoors. JD was happy removing her glasses for near, and her near acuity was 20/20 with each eye. She previously had tried multifocal lenses, but felt disoriented while wearing them. Each year JD returns for her annual examination and had relatively little change in refraction.

This year is different. JD has been experiencing ophthalmic auras without migraine. Her blood pressure is under control, although she now takes Lotrel, a different medication. She still takes Lorazepam for panic attacks, which have been increasing in frequency. During the past year, she was treated for a basal cell carcinoma on her nose, understandably adding to her anxiety. JD notes blur at distance with her glasses and feels insecure about driving at night.

Lensometry
OD: –1.50 –0.50 × 10
OS: –1.50 –0.50 × 160

Objective

Ocular Health Assessment
N/E

Clinical Measures

	At 20 ft (6 m)	At 16 in. (40 cm)
VA (sc):	OD: 20/50 (6/15)	20/25 (6/7.5)
	OS: 20/50 (6/15)	20/25 (6/7.5)
Cover Test:	Sl exop	Sl exop
N.P.C.:	N/E	
Retinoscopy/	OD: –1.00 –1.25 × 30	
Autorefractor:	OS: –1.50 –2.00 × 156	
Subjective:	OD: –1.00 –1.00 × 30	VA 20/20 (6/6)
	OS: –1.00 –1.50 × 160	VA 20/20 (6/6)

	At 20 ft (6 m)	*At 16 in. (40 cm)*
Phoria:	Ortho	3 exop
Base-in vergences:	N/E	N/E
Base-out vergences:	N/E	N/E
Accom. Amplitude:	N/E	
Neg. Rel. Accom.:	N/E	
Pos. Rel. Accom.:	N/E	
Fused X-Cyl.:	+2.25	
Stereo:	N/E	

Assessment

Compound myopic astigmatism OU and presbyopia.

Plan

1. Based on trial framing, we decide to prescribe the subjective finding in single-vision form for distance, advising her to continue removing her glasses for reading.
2. We follow **clinical pearl 18**, which is a reminder to advise all patients that there may be an adjustment period when they first start wearing their new prescription.
3. JD returns, stating that she cannot describe her problem exactly. However, she notices that, when she is sitting down looking straight ahead, everything seems fine. As soon as she looks around or begins to walk, things feel disturbing.
4. JD has used her own frame to fill the new prescription, so a change in frame size or shape is not a factor. We check the base curves, PDs, lens material, pantoscopic angle, and adjustment of the glasses; no variable seems to account for the difficulty she is having. We repeat the refraction and come up with findings similar to JD's previous subjective refraction.

We mention to JD that the new prescription does not seem to be that different from the prescription we gave her last year. She sheepishly tells us that she had been unable to wear those glasses also but was too embarrassed to tell us. Looking back in her file, the prescription written was

OD: −1.00 −1.00 × 20
OS: −1.25 −1.00 × 160

    With the emphasis her medical history warranted during JD's examination, I had not noticed that the glasses my assistant neutralized as JD's current glasses did not match the power that I had prescribed most recently. Had I glanced at that, I would have asked her why she was not wearing her most recent prescription. By assuming that JD had adapted well to the cylindrical increase made the previous year, I assumed she would have no problem adjusting to a further increase in cylinder and change in axis. The outcome of JD's case was that we remade the prescription in the following power:

OD: −1.25 −0.75 × 20
OS: −1.25 −0.75 × 160

    The new power is close enough to what she was wearing that she perceived some increase in clarity with no adaptive difficulty.

Recalcitrant Refractive Cases

Sometimes it seems like the patient is being unreasonable but has difficulty in adapting despite everyone's best intentions. Certainly **clinical pearl 20** applies in many cases of inability to adapt to cylindrical changes. When the patient brings in a bag of previous eyewear that he or she was unable to adapt to, we are very likely to add to the collection.

    The patient who does not have to wear prescriptive lenses full time usually has more difficulty adapting to a change in prescription. For example, a patient with low to moderate hyperopic astigmatism may wear the lenses only when working on the computer. A patient with low to moderate myopic astigmatism may use the prescription only for driving. Therefore, each time the patient puts on the eyewear he or she has to make the spatial adaptation to the change in cylinder power or axis all over again. This is more disconcerting than for the patient who wears glasses from the moment he or she arises until bedtime. Simply reassuring the patient that he or she will adapt to the new prescription often works, but it is not an absolute remedy. Keep in mind **clinical pearl 15**, that the patient's last doctor may be wiser than you initially realized, particularly when it comes to underprescribing cylinder or modifying cylinder axis to be less oblique.

Despite advanced planning and due consideration to clinical pearls, even expert refractionists are going to have patients who cannot adjust to the change in their prescription. If you have taken into account the probable sources of the patients' adaptive difficulty and they still complain about the prescription, it often pays to cut your losses. This usually involves remaking the lenses in a power very close to what the patient had been wearing. On rare occasions we encounter patients who claim not to be able to adapt to what we prescribe, even if we make an exact duplicate of what they previously had. In time, we learn not to take these cases personally and move on. The patient likely will become someone else's refractive challenge.

References

1. Duke-Elder S. *The Practice of Refraction*, 7th ed. St. Louis: Mosby, 1963:94.
2. Milder B, Rubin ML. *The Fine Art of Prescribing Glasses without Making a Spectacle of Yourself*, 2nd ed. Gainesville, FL: Triad Scientific Publishers, 1991:78.
3. Newman JM. Analysis, interpretation and prescription for the ametropias and heterophorias. In: WJ Benjamin (ed). *Borish's Clinical Refraction*. Philadelphia: Saunders, 1998:793–800.
4. Capone RC. Astigmatism. In: KE Brookman (ed). *Refractive Management of Ametropia*. Boston: Butterworth–Heinemann, 1996:78.
5. Borish IM. *Clinical Refraction*, 3rd ed. Chicago: Professional Press, 1970:139–140.
6. Forrest EB. A new model for functional astigmatism. *J Am Optom Assoc.* 1981;52:889–897.
7. Werner DL. Ethics in the optometric curriculum. *J Optom Educ.* 1996;21:124–125.

8. Capone RC. Astigmatism. In: KE Brookman (ed). *Refractive Management of Ametropia*. Boston: Butterworth–Heinemann, 1996:83–84.

9. Ciuffreda KJ, Levi DM, Selenow A. *Amblyopia: Basic and Clinical Aspects*. Boston: Butterworth–Heinemann, 1991:58.

10. Ingram RM. Refraction as a means of predicting squint or amblyopia in preschool siblings of children known to have these defects. *Br J Ophthalmol*. 1979;63:228.

11. Garzia RP. Management of amblyopia in infants, toddlers, and preschool children. *Problems in Optometry*. 1990;2(3):439.

12. Ciner EB. Refractive error in young children: Evaluation and prescription. *Practical Optometry*. 1992;3:182–190.

13. Press LJ. *Applied Concepts in Vision Therapy*. St. Louis: Mosby, 1997:78.

14. Birnbaum MH. Functional relationship between myopia, accommodative stress, and against-the-rule astigmia: A hypothesis. *J Am Optom Assoc*. 1978;49:911–914.

15. Grosvenor T, Quintero S, Perrigin D. Predicting refractive astigmatism: A suggested simplification of Javal's rule. *Am J Optom Physiol Opt*. 1988;65:292–297.

CHAPTER 6

Meeting the Challenges
of the Presbyopic Patient

For many patients, particularly those who pride themselves in maintaining health and longevity, presbyopia is the first loss of function associated with age. It is disconcerting. To the doctor it may simply be nature's first gentle tap of mortality, but the patient wonders, Is this a harbinger of things to come?

> Suddenly you're fifty;
> if you know anything about steps
> you're playing chess
> with an old, complicated friend.
>
> But you're walking to a schoolyard
> where kids are playing full-court,
> telling yourself the value of experience,
>
> a worn down basketball under your arm,
> your legs hanging from your waist
> like misplaced sloths in a country
> known for its cheetahs and its sunsets.[1]

Presbyopia is defined as a reduction in accommodative amplitude normally occurring with age, with onset typically around the age of 40 years.[2] Its uniqueness in the realm of refractive care is that it is the only refractive condition guaranteed to be experienced by every patient who lives long enough, although there are interventions on the horizon that may be able to alter the process.

Announcing itself as a gradual but rude awakening to the aging process, the highest incidence of presbyopia is the onset of near blur in persons ages 42 to 44.[3] The prevalence of the condition is close to 100% of the population over the age of 40.[4] The onset of presbyopia depends on a number of variables, including

- Amplitude of accommodation.
- Amount of accommodation comfortably available.
- Habitual working and reading distances.
- Physiognomy (length of arms and posture).
- Size of pupil (depth of focus).

Patients therefore may be unaware of near-point blur if they reflexively hold material farther away, do their principal near work at a computer, have low to moderate uncorrected myopia in one or both eyes, work in conditions of optimal lighting, have physiologically small pupils, or take medication that constricts the pupils.

The blurring of small print at near generally is noticed around age 40 for a specific reason. As a rule of thumb, near print should be comfortable as long as one half the amplitude of accommodation can be kept in reserve,[5] although others have suggested one third as the minimum amount of accommodation to be kept in reserve to maintain comfort and clarity.[6] Therefore, if the patient is reading at a distance of 40 cm with an accommodative demand of 2.5 diopters, the amount of accommodation in reserve should be at least 2.5 diopters (according to the one-half rule), for a total of 5 diopters. According to most authorities, the limit of 5 diopters of accommodative amplitude occurs around age 40. Table 6-1 is Donder's table for accommodative amplitude predicted as a function of age.

Several biological factors contribute to age-related presbyopic changes, principally related to changes in the crystalline lens, ciliary muscle anatomy, and possibly in choroidal elasticity. These factors are reviewed in detail elsewhere and play no role in deriving prescriptions for the patient with presbyopia.[7] The age-

Table 6-1   Donder's Table

Age (years)	Amplitude (D)
35	5.50
40	4.50
45	3.50
50	2.50
55	1.75
60	1.00
65	0.50

Table 6-2   Approximate Add Predicted by Age

Age (years)	Approximate Add (D)
40–44	+0.75 to +1.00
45–49	+1.00 to +1.50
50–54	+1.50 to +1.75
55–57	+1.75 to +2.00
58–61	+2.00 to +2.50
62–65+	+2.50 to +3.00 and higher

Source: Adapted from Eskridge JB, Amos JF, Bartlett JD. *Clinical Procedures in Optometry*. Philadelphia: Lippincott, 1991.

related changes in presbyopia are universal enough to permit the prediction of add values based on age. These are the values used to calculate over-the-counter readers and can be useful as a starting point in knowing what to expect a patient to require for near-point clarity. As stressed earlier, this is only a starting point and there is no guarantee that an individual patient will require a specific add value based on age (Table 6-2).

Some Paradoxes of Presbyopia

Although blur at near is the hallmark of presbyopia, distance blur can be associated with the condition as well. Many early presbyopes report that, in addition to blur at near, they have difficulty refocusing to distance.[8] This is an accommodative hysteresis secondary to near-point tasks. The time delay in refocusing increases with time on task as well as the intensity of the task. The delay in relaxation of accommodation after sustained near-point tasks is known as near-work-induced transient myopia (NITM). NITM is discussed more in relation to nonpresbyopic patients than presbyopic patients.[9] The premise is that, since NITM presumably is lenticular in origin, reduced accommodative ability would tend to limit or preclude a myopic aftereffect of near work.[10] However, as Milder and Rubin note, the inability to relax accommodation quickly in presbyopia is as much a manifestation of the loss of lens elasticity as the loss of accommodation itself.[8]

When patients in early presbyopia receive a plus lens addition, the demand on accommodation is lessened. The same holds true when the patient adapts by holding near-point material farther away or increases the viewing distance to a computer monitor. Consequently, when the patient refocuses to a distance, there is less accommodative response to relax. As an example, an emmetropic patient reading at 40 cm has an accommodative demand of 2.50 diopters and must relax that dioptric amount when refocusing to distance. Reading through a +1.00 add, the same patient's accommodative demand is only 1.50 diopters, and refocusing to distance requires only 1.50 diopters of accommodative relaxation. Transient distance blur after near tasks can occur in presbyopic patients with emmetropia, myopia, hyperopia, or astigmatism. This discussion does not take into consideration the patient's binocular status or the potential interaction of convergence-accommodation factors.

Patients with uncorrected or undercorrected hyperopia tend to experience the symptoms of presbyopia relatively earlier. Due to lens effectivity, myopic patients with spectacle correction tend to experience near blur relatively later, often not until age 44 or 45.[11] Patients having low to moderate myopia in one eye have natural monovision. They use their nonmyopic to see clearly at distance, and their uncorrected myopic eye to see clearly at near. These patients may not experience symptoms of presbyopia until age 50 or beyond, when the accommodative demand ultimately exceeds the amount of "built-in add" afforded by the uncorrected or undercorrected myopia. An example of this follows.

Subjective

Case History, Including Signs, Symptoms, and Visual Needs

Patient IH is a 46-year-old woman who has never worn glasses. She has never had an eye examination but now has a vision plan at work and decides to take advantage of it. IH has no visual symptoms, and her general health is reportedly fine.

Objective

Ocular Health Assessment

N/E

Clinical Measures

		At 20 ft (6 m)	At 16 in. (40 cm)
VA (no prescription):	OD:	20/20 (6/6)	20/50 (6/15)
	OS:	20/60 (6/18)	20/20 (6/15)
Cover Test:		Ortho	Sl. exop
N.P.C.:		3 in./6 in. OD out	
Retinoscopy/	OD:	Plano –0.25 × 85	
Autorefractor:	OS:	–1.25 –0.25 × 85	
Subjective:	OD:	Plano	VA 20/20 (6/6)
	OS:	–1.50 DS	VA 20/20 (6/6)
Phoria:		1 eso	3 exop
Base-in vergences:		N/E	N/E
Base-out vergences:		N/E	N/E
Accom. Amplitude:		4.50	
Neg. Rel. Accom.:		N/E	
Pos. Rel. Accom.:		N/E	
Fused X-Cyl.:		+1.50 add, giving 20/20 (6/6) in each eye at 16 in. (40 cm)	
Stereo:		N/E	

Assessment

Natural monovision, with right eye used for distance and left eye for near.

Plan

We did not give IH a lens prescription. Several factors were involved in the decision. Giving IH a prescription for driving would blur the dashboard and make it necessary to take the glasses off to view printed directions. Giving her a multifocal, with the distance prescription in the left eye and an add OU would complicate her life and also restrict the near field of view compared to her uncorrected abilities.

We counseled IH as to why she can see clearly at both distance and near without glasses. Many patients with natural monovision who have never been examined before may not realize that one eye sees better at distance and the other at near.

If we use the "half in reserve" rule, the patient should be able to see clearly at near with the left eye until the accommodative demand exceeds 3 diopters, which occurs around age 50. If we were to see IH at age 50 with these same distance findings, we would expect her to report that now she has to push small print farther away to focus clearly at near. The effective add of +1.50, obtained by not having the –1.50 prescription for the left eye, no longer is adequate for the accommodative demand. We probably would find that the X-cyl finding at near has increased to +2.00 (+0.50 as a gross lens value in the phoroptor in front of the left eye). In other words, the left eye now takes +0.50 DS to see clearly and comfortably at 16 in. (40 cm). The optimal prescription would be a single vision prescription with plano in the right eye and +0.50 in the left eye, to be used mostly for near. This would allow IH to look up or walk around with a single-vision prescription in a work environment, continuing to use the right eye for clear distance vision.

What if IH has a 46-year-old twin sister, IH-2, who has identical findings but a refraction of –0.75 DS OD and –1.50 DS OS. Unlike her twin sister, IH-2 is beginning to notice some distance blur but is happy with her uncorrected near vision. In this instance, we leave the left lens plano for near, but should we prescribe the full minus for the right eye? Generally speaking, we have better success in leaving the patient a bit underminused, preserving some intermediate clarity. The best way to determine this is to follow **clinical pearl 4** and have the patient hold the

–0.75 trial lens over the right eye while looking out the window at signs, as well as looking around the room at intermediate distances. The probability is that IH-2 will tell you that the lens feels peculiar or uncomfortable. Rather than trying to convince her otherwise, substitute a trial lens of –0.50.

Leaving the patient uncorrected or underminused in one eye is quite different from prescribing plus at near for one eye only. When a higher amount of myopia in one eye has been either present for a long time or acquired slowly, it does not present the adaptive problems that might be present with doctor-induced monovision. In fact, the doctor who prescribes lenses that interfere with natural monovision is violating **clinical pearl 14** of conventional wisdom, which advises not to try to improve upon the asymptomatic state.

Once it has been determined that the patient can benefit from a plus lens addition at near, there are various methods to determine the optimal add value. As previously mentioned, one guide is to prescribe the minimum add that would allow the patient to keep one third to one half of his or her accommodative amplitude in reserve for most near-point demands. Another rule of thumb is to prescribe the amount of plus at near that balances the NRA/PRA findings.[12] To determine the plus lens value, take the absolute difference between the higher number and the lower number and divide by 2. For example, if through the distance refraction one obtains an NRA of +2.50 and a PRA of –1.00, the add that would balance the two findings is +0.75.

Another useful rule is to derive an add based on the value that will place the patient's usual near working distance at the dioptric midpoint of the range of clear vision. This is the range in space from the nearest point at which the patient can see clearly through the add to the farthest point at which the patient can see clearly through the add. An add that requires a patient to keep half of the accommodative amplitude in reserve would achieve this goal, but clinical measurements are rarely precise enough to assure that this will occur.[13] Therefore, determine the customary near working distance and move the near-point card out and then in to confirm that the range of focus is equal in both directions. For example, if we determine that a near add at 16 in. (40 cm) provides a far range of clarity at 21 in. (53 cm), the near range of clarity should be 11 in. (28 cm).

The patient's occupational and avocational needs may indicate the need to modify what is prescribed or to prescribe more than one pair of eyewear. Detailed consideration to these issues was given by Holmes, Joliffe, and Gregg.[14] Although this book no longer is in print, the concept of taking a variety of needs into account is well recognized by clinicians. Patients engaged in a near environment with reference material spread out (such as attorneys or accountants) need a wider array of foci than an assembly line worker whose near demand is at a relatively fixed distance. Contemporary demands of the work environment often center around distances or positions of gaze unique to computer users.[15,16] Failure to recognize these needs appears in some of the cases discussed in Chapter 13, regarding the dissatisfied patient.

Clinical pearl 1, reminding us to listen to the patient, is vital in determining the near-point needs of presbyopic patients. Patients with spherical equivalents of myopia up to 3 diopters in one or both eyes often are happier in taking off their glasses for near than with a multifocal lens. The built-in magnification factor is limited by the range of focus at near when the glasses are removed. For example, the patient with 5 diopters of myopia has to maintain a near focus of approximately 8 in. (20 cm) to see small print clearly when the glasses are removed. In addition, it will probably be difficult to sustain the demands of convergence at that viewing distance, necessitating closing one eye to avoid visual fatigue or diplopia. Nevertheless, avoid the temptation of violating **clinical pearl 14**. If the patient tells you he or she feels fine by simply taking off the glasses periodically to see at near, do not try to convince him or her otherwise. This is evident in the case of patient NP.

Subjective

Case History, Including Signs, Symptoms, and Visual Needs

NP, a 47-year-old systems analyst, presents for routine examination. She scheduled an appointment after receiving a reminder letter that 1 year had passed since her last examination. NP feels her distance acuity is unchanged, and the only time she is conscious of near blur is when looking at small print such as package inserts for pharmaceuticals.

Lensometry
OU: –4.00 DS

Objective

Ocular Health Assessment
There is no evidence of ocular pathology. Dilated fundus examination shows no holes, breaks, or tears.

Clinical Measures

	At 20 ft (6 m)	*At 16 in. (40 cm)*
VA (cc):	OD: 20/20 (6/6)	20/25 (6/7.5)
	OS: 20/20 (6/6)	20/25 (6/7.5)
Cover Test:	Ortho	Ortho
N.P.C.:	To the nose	
Retinoscopy/	OD: –4.25 –0.25 × 175	
Autorefractor:	OS: –4.00 –0.50 × 180	
Subjective:	OD: –4.00 DS	VA 20/20 (6/6)
	OS: –4.00 DS	VA 20/20 (6/6)
Phoria:	N/E	
Base-in vergences:	N/E	N/E
Base-out vergences:	N/E	N/E
Accom. Amplitude:	4.00	
Neg. Rel. Accom.:	+2.25	
Pos. Rel. Accom.:	–1.50	
Fused X-Cyl.:	+0.50 add, giving 20/20 (6/6) in each eye at 16 in. (40 cm)	
Stereo:	N/E	

Assessment

This patient has stable myopia. Her increasing presbyopic demands still can be met by removing her glasses for near, and she does not seem inconvenienced in doing this.

Plan

We do not change the patient's prescription. We demonstrate that there are new multifocal lens types that would allow her to keep her eyewear on for most near work. After pointing out the relative advantages, we acknowledge that a compromise must be made in both the functional field of view and the magnification provided. Note that, as a systems analyst, NP spends a good deal of her day on the computer. Her relatively remote working distance coupled with a higher accommodative amplitude than what you would expect for her age, allows her to use her distance prescription comfortably most of the day. At select times, when she needs to see fine print as on prescription labels or maps, she sees adequately by removing her eyewear and holding the material at 10 in. (25 cm). She needs to do this only briefly, so the demand on her binocular vision is not an issue, or she closes one eye for a moment. Newspaper print can be managed with acuity as low as 20/50 (6/15), and NP still handles that with no problem at a normal reading distance through her single-vision glasses. She does not want to complicate her life with a multifocal or with multiple prescriptions, and there is no need to do so at present.

Pearls and Perils of Presbyopia

As evidenced by the preceding discussion, patients bring a host of factors to presbyopia that cause the doctor to temper what is being prescribed or at least to offer the patient several options. Here, we survey some of the factors specific to the various phases and states of presbyopia.

Phase 1: Early Presbyopia

Patients initially experiencing presbyopia usually have more difficulty with near vision than distance vision. If the patient has myopia, first check to see if the distance refraction shows less minus than the habitual prescription. Reducing distance minus is equivalent to giving the patient plus power at near and may delay the need for multiple prescription powers. Such was the case with patient DW.

Subjective

Case History, Including Signs, Symptoms, and Visual Needs

DW is a 43-year-old cardiologist who notices lately that he's having trouble focusing at near. He has always been the picture of health and cannot believe he is starting to take his glasses off when looking at small print. He would like to know if there is anything he can do to avoid wearing bifocals.

Lensometry
OU: –2.50 DS

Objective

Ocular Health Assessment
N/E

Clinical Measures

	At 20 ft (6 m)	At 16 in. (40 cm)
VA (cc):	OD: 20/20 (6/6)	20/25 (6/7.5)
	OS: 20/20 (6/6)	20/25 (6/7.5)
Cover Test:	Sl esop	Ortho
N.P.C.:	To the nose	
Retinoscopy/	OD: –2.00 –0.25 × 100	
Autorefractor:	OS: –2.00 –0.25 × 80	
Subjective:	OD: –2.00 DS	VA 20/20 (6/6)
	OS: –2.00 DS	VA 20/20 (6/6)
Phoria:	Ortho	4 exop
Base-in vergences:	N/E	N/E
Base-out vergences:	N/E	N/E
Accom. Amplitude:	5.00	
Neg. Rel. Accom.:	+2.25	
Pos. Rel. Accom.:	–1.75	
Fused X-Cyl.:	+0.50 Add, giving 20/20 in each eye at 16 in.	
Stereo:	N/E	

Assessment

Myopia OU, reduced from previous examination. We confirmed with trial lenses that DW could see slightly better with less minus at distance, and this reduction also improves clarity for small print at near.

Plan

We prescribe new single-vision glasses for use at distance and near. We counsel the patient that he is fortunate that there is a simple solution to his visual needs at this time but a multifocal prescription or removing his glasses for small print is inevitable in the future.

DW is fortunate that his distance myopia had lessened, but the more common scenario in early presbyopia is what happened to patient LL.

Subjective

Case History, Including Signs, Symptoms, and Visual Needs

LL is a 43-year-old dentist who is beginning to have trouble focusing at near. Detecting subtle visual alterations in gums and teeth is his livelihood, and he lacks the luxury of taking off his glasses to see at near on the job, like some of his nondentist acquaintances. He mentions that, if he does need bifocals, it would not surprise him, but he would rather have lenses without a line. His hobbies include fishing and skiing, and he has no problem doing either of these with his current glasses.

Lensometry
OD: $-2.25 -0.75 \times 115$
OS: $-2.50 -0.25 \times 75$

Objective

Ocular Health Assessment
N/E

Clinical Measures

	At 20 ft (6 m)	At 16 in. (40 cm)
VA (cc):	OD: 20/20	20/25
	OS: 20/20	20/25
Cover Test:	Ortho	Sl exop
N.P.C.:	2 in./4 in. (5 cm/10 cm) OS out; no diplopia	
Retinoscopy/	OD: −2.50 −0.75 × 110	
Autorefractor:	OS: −2.75 −0.50 × 85	
Subjective:	OD: −2.50 −0.75 × 115	VA 20/20 (6/6)
	OS: −2.75 −0.25 × 75	VA 20/20 (6/6)
Phoria:	Ortho	4 exop
Base-in vergences:	N/E	N/E
Base-out vergences:	N/E	N/E
Accom. Amplitude:	5.00	
Neg. Rel. Accom.:	+2.50	
Pos. Rel. Accom.:	−1.00	
Fused X-Cyl.:	+1.00 add, giving 20/20 (6/6) in each eye at 16 in. (40 cm)	
Stereo:	N/E	

Assessment

Slight increase in myopia OU with presbyopia. On trial framing, patient preferred +0.75 at near over his habitual prescription for optimum near clarity in a simulated work environment.

Plan

1. We kept the distance prescription the same, and gave LL a progressive addition lens (PAL) with a +1.00 add.
2. We offered the option of a separate pair of occupational or avocational lenses as single vision for near only.

Note that, even though LL's distance refraction increased by −0.25 sphere, it would be counterproductive to increase distance minus in an early presbyope who has no distance complaints. This is a corollary to **clinical pearl 11**. The extra minus that is not needed at intermediate distances makes it unnecessarily more difficult to focus on objects such as the dashboard when driving, wall charts, and shelf labeling. Second, it is helpful to simulate occupational viewing distances when prescribing for near. For a computer operator, this can be done by letting the patient sit at a workstation. A dentist has a significant range of near foci, including inspecting instruments, working on teeth, reading X rays, looking at charts, and working from various distances, including sitting and standing. A progressive addition lens is ideal for a dentist's vocational requirements.

If the patient prefers to wear lined multifocal lenses, do not talk him or her out of it. Do mention that the best and easiest time to adapt to a progressive lens is in early presbyopia. The lower add powers in any design provide relatively wide and undistorted lateral fields of view. Occupational or avocational lenses can be offered, particularly for individuals who use computers for significant periods of time.

Many patients in early presbyopia present for evaluation because a spouse pushed them to have an examination or because they are feeling their mortality for the first time. The glasses you prescribe are their first "real" pair of glasses. They intuitively know that the glasses purchased in the drugstore are great as spare pairs, but that they should probably have one "workhorse" set of glasses made specifically for their eyes. They also know that they wear down one heel on their shoe faster than the other one and have learned that all paired organs in their body may not be exactly alike. When you tell them that their eyes are not exactly alike and that drugstore glasses do not take that into consideration, they are not surprised. However, they basically are happy with the drugstore glasses, see no need for a distance prescription, and do not want to complicate their lives with multifocal lenses. Such was the case for patient LS.

Subjective

Case History, Including Signs, Symptoms, and Visual Needs
LS is the 45-year-old mayor of our town, who is also a real estate broker. His visual needs are highly varied, and he never felt com-

pelled to have his eyes examined because he always had perfect vision. He confesses that he has been using drugstore reading glasses recently for woodworking, his hobby, and has several pair. For casual reading, he uses the weakest reading glasses the store had; and for woodworking, he uses a stronger pair for extra magnification.

Lensometry

+1.00 OU and +2.00 OU over-the-counter reading glasses.

Objective

Ocular Health Assessment

N/E

Clinical Measures

	At 20 ft (6 m)	At 16 in. (40 cm)
VA (sc):	OD: 20/25 (6/7.5)	20/30 (6/9)
	OS: 20/30 (6/9)	20/25 (6/7.5)
Cover Test:	Ortho	Sl exop
N.P.C.:	3 in./5 in. (7.5 cm/10 cm) OD out;	
	no diplopia	
Retinoscopy/	OD: +0.25 –0.75 × 45	
Autorefractor:	OS: +0.50 –1.00 × 135	
Subjective:	OD: Plano –0.50 × 45	VA 20/20
	OS: +0.50 –1.00 × 130	VA 20/20
Phoria:	Ortho	4 exop
Base-in vergences:	N/E	N/E
Base-out vergences:	N/E	N/E
Accom. Amplitude:	4.00	
Neg. Rel. Accom.:	+2.50	
Pos. Rel. Accom.:	–1.25	
Fused X-Cyl.:	+1.00 add, giving 20/20 (6/6) in	
	each eye at 16 in. (40 cm)	
Stereo:	N/E	

Assessment

Early presbyopia OU with mild astigmatism OU.

Plan

We prescribe single-vision near-only lenses, as follows:

OD: +1.25 –0.25 × 45
OS: +1.25 –0.50 × 135

We offer the patient the option of half-eyes or a task lens such as Readables. The possibility of PALs or a unilateral monovision contact lens is mentioned.

Several principles are in operation here. The first is **clinical pearl 5A**, which cautions against reducing net plus at near for a presbyopic patient. The patient is happy with his +1.00 drugstore readers, so if we are going to incorporate a cylindrical correction, we also have to take into account **clinical pearl 10** and note its effect on the spherical component. We want to keep the near plus effect at approximately +1.00. Therefore, in prescribing –0.25 cylinder for the right eye and –0.50 cylinder for the left eye, we also increased the plus sphere to +1.25.

You may also wonder why we cut the cylinder and prescribed only half of the power determined to provide the best clarity. Although spatial adaptation at near typically is not problematic, LS still must refocus to distance when taking off his glasses or looking above the lenses with half-eyes. Having more cylinder in the reading prescription than is necessary for the patient to be happy at near results in the feeling that distance clarity requires more effort than before.

Clinical pearl 6 also is appropriate to mention in this case. In making an asymmetrical prescription change (we are adding more cylinder to the left eye than the patient is used to), we prefer to be conservative. The amount of cylinder added should be just enough for LS to notice that near acuity is a bit sharper if not more comfortable, yet not sufficient to cause problems in refocusing to a distance or switching to his spare pairs of readers. LS stockpiles spare over-the-counter readers in various places: next to the bed, in a pocketbook or valise, at the office, in the glove compartment, a small folding pair in jacket, and so on.

Even though it is tempting to encourage a distance prescription because we can make acuity sharper, many early presbyopes pride themselves on not having to wear glasses all the time. Only if LS preferred a full lens would we consider incorporating a distance prescription, in which case we might give the following prescription:

OD: Plano –0.25 × 45/ +1.25
OS: +0.25 –0.50 × 130/ +1.25

The early presbyope who should be easy to satisfy but often proves difficult is the patient with previously uncorrected or undercorrected hyperopia. **Clinical pearl 7** takes this into account in advising never to prescribe more plus power at distance than is consistent with good distance vision and comfort. This is illustrated in the case of MFP, the presbyope who mistook her husband for a wise man.

Subjective

Case History, Including Signs, Symptoms, and Visual Needs
MFP is the wife of one of the authors. MFP has a history of esotropia as a child, confirmed by family photographs. She has no recollection of visual problems as a child, and periodic examinations as an adult show low hyperopia in both eyes without the need for compensation and 20/20 (6/6) unaided acuity at distance and near with good fusion. MFP's jobs always involve considerable near work, first as a legal secretary in a large firm and ultimately as an optometric office manager. At age 40, MFP crossed the threshold of asymptomatic near vision. She recalls this happening to both her parents, who never needed glasses until her husband prescribed lenses for them. She is concerned that she may "unravel" the way they did and wind up wearing glasses full time. She, too, plans on blaming the doctor in the event that this happens.

Objective

Ocular Health Assessment
N/E

Clinical Measures

	At 20 ft (6 m)	At 16 in. (40 cm)
VA (sc):	OD: 20/20 (6/6)	20/25+ (6/7.5+)
	OS: 20/20 (6/6)	20/25+ (6/7.5+)
Cover Test:	Sl esop	Sl esop
N.P.C.:	3 in./5 in. (7.5 cm/12.5 cm) limited by blur	
Retinoscopy/	OD: +1.00 −0.25 × 90	
Autorefractor:	OS: +1.25 −0.25 × 90	
Subjective:	OD: +0.50 −0.25 × 90	VA 20/20 (6/6)
	OS: +0.75 −0.25 × 90	VA 20/20 (6/6)
Phoria:	3 esop	4 esop
Base-in vergences:	X/08/04	X/19/13
Base-out vergences:	X/14/10	X/20/12
Accom. Amplitude:	5.00	
Neg. Rel. Accom.:	+1.75	
Pos. Rel. Accom.:	−1.75	
Fused X-Cyl.:	Plano	
Stereo:	40 seconds of arc	

Assessment

Early presbyopia OU with latent hyperopia.

Plan

We prescribe +0.75 −0.25 × 90 OU; and MFP is advised that, although the glasses are intended primarily for near, she may find them beneficial for television viewing or driving.

Things work out nicely when the patient is able to tolerate looking across the room or walking about with a near prescription. **Clinical pearl 16** indicates the importance of advising the patient on what to expect with the new lenses, and it seemed reasonable to expect that MFP would have no problem adapting to this rather mild prescription. When MFP put on her beautiful new eyewear, **clinical pearl 19** came to mind. This is the one advising a practitioner to refer close relatives to distant colleagues. With her reading prescription in place, MFP promptly became queasy and announced that she could not wear the glasses. We encourage her to try them again and reassure her that she would adapt. It took awhile before she found the advice reassuring.

Clinical pearl 7 also proved to be pertinent in MFP's case. In an attempt to ease her transition into plus lenses, we decide to implement some "plus lens acceptance" vision therapy, particularly because of the esophoria and latent hyperopia.[17] This proves of little help, as attempts at accommodative rock and similar therapies only make MFP more queasy. Bearing in mind **clinical pearls 2 and 9** and the implications of small changes for sensitive patients, we reduce the prescription to +0.50 sph OU.

It took awhile, but MFP finally eased herself into the prescription for near work. She gradually found less need to take the glasses off when refixating to distance or walking about. Ultimately, she found herself at times forgetting to take her glasses off. Predictably she blamed the doctor for the situation, no longer being able to read small print in menus without her glasses whereas before she could do so with some effort. In cases such as MFP's, prescription changes should be made in small increments. Stay with single-vision lens power as long as possible. Be very cautious about multifocals, particularly PALs, until the patient has demonstrated enough visual flexibility.

Newer PAL lens designs continually chip away at the optical challenges of balancing binocular viewing and reducing lateral distortion and swim. However, two optical properties of PALs, common to all designs, can pose a clinical challenge when trying to convert a patient to progressives. It is particularly vexing when the patient had been asymptomatic with a single-vision near lens or a lined bifocal. Consider the patient who has been successfully wearing the follow prescription in a flat-top (FT-28) form:

OD: $-1.50 -0.50 \times 90/ +1.25$
OS: $-2.00 -2.00 \times 180/ +1.25$

The patient has -1.50 D of power in the vertical meridian of the right eye but -4.00 D of power in the vertical meridian of the left eye, resulting in 2.50 D of anisometropia when looking downward. The line on an FT-28 is set 3 to 4 mm below the optical center. If we allow that most reading will occur another 4 mm below the seg line, or a total of 7–8 mm below the optical center, Prentice's rule results in a vertical prism demand of 1.75–2.00 prism diopters. That is within the vertical vergence range of most presbyopes, and when it is not, slab-off prism is an option. However, because of the progressive nature of PAL optics, the full add power typically occurs 12–14 mm below the optical center, which will induce 3.00–3.50 prism diopters of vertical imbalance, which would be taxing to the vertical vergence range of most presbyopes.

A final paradox involving multifocal lenses is the prism thinning process used to improve the cosmetic appearance of the add. It is standard practice with PALs and induces prism base down in each lens. The value of the base-down prism is directly linked to the add power and is approximately two thirds of the add power in diopters (Table 6-3).

Prism that occurs in the same base direction in both eyes is known as *yoked prism*. Although the values we deal with here are relatively small, the amount of yoked prism prescribed that sometimes effects behavioral changes is relatively small.[18] The point to

Table 6-3   Prism Thinning in Varilux Progressive Addition Lenses

Varilux Addition	BD Prism (D)
0.75	0.5
1.00	
1.25	0.75
1.50	1.00
1.75	
2.00	1.25
2.25	1.50
2.50	
2.75	1.75
3.00	2.00
3.25	
3.50	2.25

Source: Data from Varilux Corporation, 2000, *Product Guide*, LPAN200009.

be emphasized is that the induced yoked prism base-down effect in PALs can contribute to adaptive symptoms, particularly when moving a patient into a higher add power who has not previously used a PAL. It is another reason to start patients in PALs when their add requirements are relatively low, so that changes occurring in lens optics as the add increases require minimal adaptation.

Phase 2: Basic Presbyopia

As the patient progresses further into presbyopia, clarity at intermediate distances becomes a concern. We continue the discussion regarding the patient who manifests increasing hyperopia. If we take the preceding case, eventually MFP's requirement for plus at near will exceed what she can tolerate at distance. When moving into a multifocal lens, it will be advantageous to put the maximum amount of plus that is tolerated into the distance portion of the lens. The main reason for doing this is that the patient will have additional plus power for intermediate viewing distances before having to dip into the PAL corridor. We now look at patient MFP's numbers at age 45.

Subjective

Case History, Including Signs, Symptoms, and Visual Needs

Since her first prescription 5 years ago, which was +0.50 sph OU, MFP has progressed to +1.00 sph OU. Although she uses the glasses primarily for near and intermediate distances, there are times where she finds herself driving with them simply because she forgets to take them off. When she removes the glasses, she still feels that she sees fine, although she loathes driving at night, with or without glasses. Antireflective coating on the lenses has made no difference with her aversion to night driving. Occasionally, MFP helps out in the dispensing area of the office and uses +2.00 half-eyes to see the small numbers imprinted on frames. She notes that, at home or in restaurants, where the lighting is not as bright as in the office, she struggles at near with the +1.00 prescription.

Objective

Ocular Health Assessment

N/E

Clinical Measures

		At 20 ft (6 m)	At 16 in. (40 cm)
VA (sc):	OD:	20/20 (6/6)	20/30+ (6/7.5+)
	OS:	20/20 (6/6)	20/30+ (6/7.5+)
Cover Test:		Sl esop	Sl esop
N.P.C.:		4 in./6 in. (10 cm/15 cm) limited by blur	
Retinoscopy/	OD:	+1.50 –0.25 × 85	
Autorefractor:	OS:	+1.50 –0.25 × 95	
Subjective:	OD:	+1.50 –0.25 × 90	VA 20/20 (6/6)
	OS:	+1.50 –0.25 × 90	VA 20/20 (6/6)
Phoria:		2 esop	4 esop
Base-in vergences:		X/08/04	X/19/13
Base-out vergences:		X/14/10	X/20/12
Accom. Amplitude:		5.00	
Neg. Rel. Accom.:		+2.25	
Pos. Rel. Accom.:		–1.00	
Fused X-Cyl.:		+1.25	
Stereo:		40 seconds of arc	

Assessment

Basic presbyopia OU with increasingly manifest hyperopia.

Plan

We propose a PAL with prescription, +1.25 sph OU/+1.00 add, and demonstrate the PAL to the patient before ordering.

MFP presently wears a +1.00 single-vision prescription and needs more plus at near. We could increase her distance prescription by +0.25, and this would likely placate her for another 6 months. However, she no longer is the sensitive presbyope alluded to in **clinical pearl 9**, and her variety of near-point demands has earned her the right to a lens with greater flexibility.

In some instances, when the patient is perfectly happy with distance vision, it is a mistake to push plus at distance. However, in the case of the unraveling hyperopic presbyope, prescribing the maximum plus accepted comfortably at distance minimizes the amount of the add. Irrespective of which progressive lens is selected, peripheral distortion increases with increasing add power. Therefore, putting as much plus in the distance as possible enables the practitioner to use a lesser add power and, therefore, keep peripheral distortion to a minimum. This is particularly advantageous when easing a visually sensitive patient, like MFP, into her first add. When selecting a frame with a small vertical (B) dimension, transferring as much plus as can be accepted into the distance portion lessens the need for the patient to get to the bottom of the lens before locating adequate plus for most tasks (Figure 6-1).

Bear in mind that, by increasing the distance portion by just +0.25, MFP will experience increased clarity for printing on shelves (as in the supermarket) and in her computer workstation environment. When searching for small optical details or reading a menu in a dimly lit restaurant, the +0.75 or +1.00 portion of the PAL will circumvent the need for a separate near prescription of higher plus power.

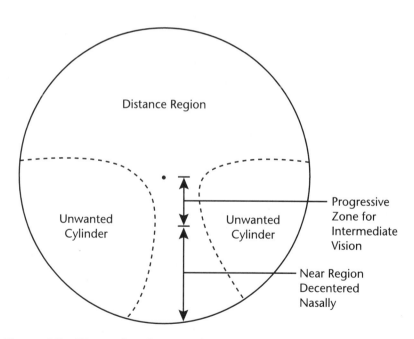

Figure 6-1   The optics of a generic progressive addition lens. (Reprinted from Brooks CW, Borish IM. *System for Ophthalmic Dispensing,* **2nd ed. Boston: Butterworth–Heinemann, 1996:296.)**

It is easiest to adapt to a PAL with a relatively low add power because peripheral distortion is kept to a minimum. Always prescribe the lowest add power necessary for the patient's habitual working distance.[19] We encourage emerging presbyopes to obtain a PAL prescription as soon as it becomes evident that they need a multifocal. Even with the softest designs, some patients determined to avoid lined bifocals will not be able to adapt to a PAL. For some a PAL will provide insufficient width in the near portion of the lens. When the patient is not yet in need of an intermediate prescription and simply wants to avoid the line in a flat-top bifocal, the alternative to a PAL is a blended 28 bifocal (Figure 6-2). The caveat in using a blended 28 is that the transition zone between distance and near creates an arc or band of distortion several millimeters in height. However, this region is uniform and some find it easier to function with than a PAL.

We have devoted significant attention to the patient with hyperopia who gradually accepts more plus at distance as well as near. Next we return to the patient with myopia who is advancing to the next stage of presbyopia. We look again at patient NP, introduced earlier in the section on paradoxes in presbyopia.

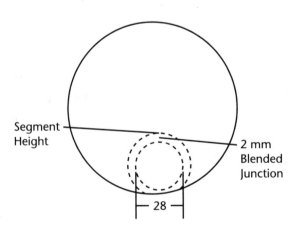

Figure 6-2   The optics of a blended 28 bifocal lens.

Subjective

Case History, Including Signs, Symptoms, and Visual Needs

When we left patient NP, she was a 47-year-old systems analyst who had sufficient accommodation for her age to function well at near point through her –4.00 DS OU glasses. She removed her eyewear for small print as needed. NP now is 50 years old and reports that, although her distance acuity is unchanged, she no longer can function effectively at near through her glasses. She has been removing them at times and getting closer to the computer screen, but this is impractical when she needs to do training and because it constrains her work space.

Lensometry
OU –4.00 DS

Objective

Ocular Health Assessment
N/E

Clinical Measures

	At 20 ft (6 m)	At 16 in. (40 cm)
VA (cc):	OD: 20/20 (6/6)	20/40 (6/12)
	OS: 20/20 (6/6)	20/40 (6/12)
Cover Test:	Ortho	Ortho
N.P.C.:	4 in./6 in. (10 cm/15 cm), limited by blur	
Retinoscopy/	OD: –4.00 –0.25 × 170	
Autorefractor:	OS: –4.00 –0.25 × 180	
Subjective:	OD: –4.00 DS	VA 20/20
	OS –4.00 DS	VA 20/20
Phoria:	N/E	
Base-in vergences:	N/E	N/E
Base-out vergences:	N/E	N/E
Accom. Amplitude:	3 D OD/OS	
Neg. Rel. Accom.:	+2.75	
Pos. Rel. Accom.:	–0.50	

Fused X-Cyl.:	+1.75 add, giving 20/20 (6/6) in each eye at 16 in. (40 cm)
Stereo:	N/E

Assessment

NP has increased presbyopia with stable myopia. Her near-point demands no longer are met totally through her distance prescription or by removing her glasses for near.

Plan

We prescribe a PAL prescription, offering the additional options of a task-specific bifocal prescription as well as a task-specific single-vision near prescription.

A progressive addition lens offers the most flexibility in selecting the appropriate power for various near-point demands. If NP proceeds with a PAL prescription, a good starting point would be –4.00 DS OU/+1.50. This amount of plus at near should be sufficient for computer and general reading tasks. We might even begin with less of an add. As reviewed earlier, higher PAL add power provides more magnification but further restricts the useful field of view at near. It is important to remind the patient at dispensing that there still will be times when she might feel the need to remove her glasses for small print and that magnification will be significantly greater than what she will experience through the maximum portion of her add.

Patient NP has several options to consider. If the optics of a PAL do not afford a wide enough area for viewing the computer and other task needs, she can switch to a bifocal prescription. If NP has the need to refocus to distance often (for example, seeing projected presentations at client meetings), she may do well with a prescription of –4.00 DS OU/+1.50 and a relatively high seg for comfortable computer viewing through the add. If most of her day is consumed by computer work, she may be better served by a single-vision prescription of –2.50 sph OU for use at the computer or an occupational mutifocal lens. The AO Technica, Zeiss Gradal RD, and Sola Access are some of the more popular computer task lens designs in progressive or graduated form. These lenses provide optimal focal power for standard desktop com-

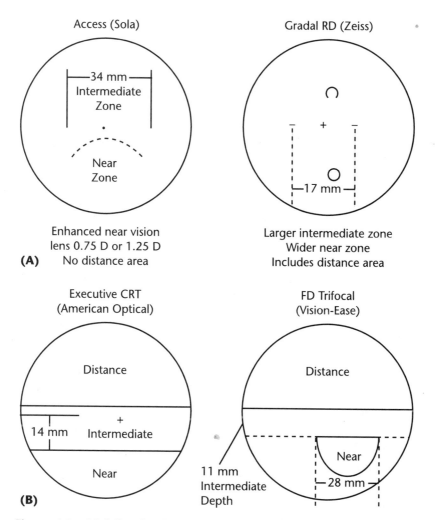

Figure 6-3   **Multifocal task lenses for computer use: A, Special-range progressive; B, Full-range trifocal.**

puter screen viewing and a continuum of power extending the focal range from near when gazing downward to mid-range distance when looking slightly upward (Figure 6-3A).*

---

*Occupational multifocals have become rather sophisticated, and it is best to consult a current reference for available options. One of the better sources for this information is the annual *Ophthalmic Lens Desk Reference,* published as a supplement to the journal *Optometric Management* each fall. Another excellent reference is the "Frames" catalog (www.FRAMESdata.com), which issues an annual lens product guide.

. An option NP probably does not need yet is an intermediate/near combination, where the carrier is used for computer viewing and the lower area is for reading small print. A final lens option, which may be more of a necessity in advanced presbyopia, is an occupational trifocal available for computer use, which affords an intermediate seg as high as 14 mm and a width to 35 mm (Figure 6-3B).

Phase 3: Advanced Presbyopia

By the time patients arrive at advanced presbyopia, they have a firm grasp of visual needs and ranges. In line with our clinical pearl of "if it ain't broke don't fix it," be mindful of preserving the patient's relative seg height if it has been working fine. For example, if the patient has a bifocal that is 4 mm below the lower lid level, which is lower than you normally set it, but is happy with the placement there, don't try to convince him or her that it needs to be higher. And if you are taking a measurement for a new frame for that patient, remember to measure the seg height again for what would result in the line being 4 mm below the lower lid (Figure 6-4).

In advanced presbyopia, **clinical pearl 5**, which advises not to reduce net plus at near when the patient is happy with near vision, is crucial. We consider the case of patient HC, who has made an appointment in response to a recall letter reminding him that it is time for his routine, comprehensive eye examination. For the moment, we suspend our template for case presentation to consider the patient's habitual prescription and subjective refraction.

HC, a 60-year-old insurance sales representative, has been happily wearing the same bifocal prescription for the past 5 years. He mentions that he tried several different "no-line bifocals" in the past and could never get used to them. What he has now seems to be working fine. Lensometry shows that he has +2.00 sphere OU at distance with a +2.50 flat-top 28 mm bifocal add OU. His distance visual acuity through his glasses is 20/25 (6/7.5) with right, left, and both eyes together. At near (40 cm) he has 20/20 (6/6) with each eye through the bifocal portion of his lenses. Refraction shows that HC's distance prescription has lessened to +1.25 sphere OU to

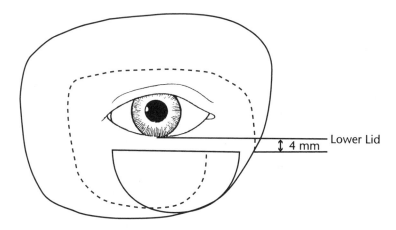

Figure 6-4 Preserving the patient's habitual relative seg height. The patient habitually likes the seg height 4 mm below the lower lid. Dashed lines represent the outline of the new, smaller frame selected. The seg height again should be specified at 4 mm below the lower lid. You may wish to advise the patient that the bifocal area will be of relatively smaller total area.

obtain a crisp 20/20 (6/6) acuity. Over the distance refraction, HC now takes a +3.25 add for best subjective acuity at 40 cm.

You might be tempted to reduce HC's distance prescription. A 60-year-old patient will enjoy hearing that his vision actually is improving at distance. But, would it be wise to reduce a distance hyperopic power when the patient is asymptomatic? We suggest that it is not, and here is why. In maintaining the +2.00 prescription at distance, HC actually has an intermediate power of +0.75. Any amount of plus at distance that you lessen is going to rob him of that intermediate clarity, such as he enjoys now when looking at his car's instrument panel, store shelves, and so on.

If you agree with this decision, we caution against demonstrating to HC that you can improve his distance acuity by reducing the power of his lenses. If you do such a demonstration, HC will probably second-guess your decision not to change his prescription. You will have to explain why reducing the power of his distance prescription will reduce the intermediate clarity he enjoys, and that usually just confuses the issue. At age 60, HC will be happy just to hear that he is doing fine and that it is unnecessary to make any changes in power at this time. If you succumb to the temptation to fiddle with his distance prescription and reduce it to +1.75 sphere OU at distance, be sure to keep the net plus at near the same and increase the add to +2.75 sphere OU.

We turn our attention to a case that strings together a few different pearls. **Clinical pearls 9 and 10** advise to be mindful of the implications of the spherocylindrical equivalent in presbyopia, and **clinical pearl 11** accentuates the importance of understanding the patient's visual needs.

Subjective

Case History, Including Signs, Symptoms, and Visual Needs

Patient LC is the 56-year-old spouse of a loquacious, long-time patient, WC. WC finally convinced his wife, who had no prior eye examination and is happy with drugstore readers, to see you because she "isn't getting any younger." In her words, everything has been falling apart. Although she does not feel her vision is bad, she has been getting tired more easily when reading, even though she uses the strongest drugstore glasses. She is a voracious reader, which allows her to tune out her husband's incessant chatter.

Lensometry

OU +3.00 over-the-counter readers

Objective

Ocular Health Assessment

Anterior chambers clear OU, pupils normal, trace cataracts OU, and vitreoretinal structures normal OU.

Clinical Measures

	At 20 ft (6 m) sc	At 16 in. (40 cm) cc
VA:	OD: 20/25 –2	20/25
	OS: 20/30 +2	20/30
Cover Test:	Ortho	6 exop
N.P.C.:	4 in./7 in. (10 cm/18 cm), limited by blur	

	At 20 ft (6 m) sc	*At 16 in. (40 cm) cc*
Retinoscopy/	OD: +0.50 −1.50 × 75	
Autorefractor:	OS: +0.75 −2.00 × 95	
Subjective:	OD: +0.50 −1.50 × 75	VA 20/20 (6/6)
	OS: +0.75 −2.00 × 95	VA 20/20 (6/6)
Phoria:	Ortho	5 exop
Base-in vergences:	N/E	X/18/12
Base-out vergences:	N/E	X/18/10
Accom. Amplitude:	1.50	
Neg. Rel. Accom.:	+2.75	
Pos. Rel. Accom.:	Plano	
Fused X-Cyl.:	+2.75 add, giving 20/20 in each eye at 16 in.	
Stereo:	40 seconds of arc	

Assessment

LC has mixed astigmatism and advanced presbyopia. Her cataracts are minimal and do not contribute to her symptoms. The drugstore readers lack an astigmatic correction that would help focusing.

Plan

1. One option is to prescribe single-vision lenses for near only,
   OD: +3.25 −1.50 × 75
   OS: +3.50 −2.00 × 95
   However, the spherical equivalent of this is only +2.50 sph OU, and the patient has been used to more magnification at +3.00 sph OU. Therefore, we trial frame the tentative prescription to make sure that the patient is both comfortable with the cylinder and happy with the net plus effect at near.
2. The best result is derived with the following prescription:
   OD: +3.50 −1.00 × 75
   OS: +3.75 −1.50 × 95
   Even though the new tentative prescription has the same spherical equivalent as the +3.00 over-the-counter readers, the fact that the cylinder is incorporated should reduce the asthenopic symptoms. As noted in **clinical pearl 9**, it is

reasonable to expect a change of 0.50 D or higher to be significant in reducing asthenopia, as long we do not reduce the net plus lens effect at near.

LC's case offers other possible prescriptive scenarios. Assume that, when you had the distance refraction in the phoropter, LC commented on how sharp everything was. On reflection, she thought that perhaps television viewing has not appeared as effortless as before. She also notices the compulsion to move closer to the screen when proofreading text. When you suggest multiple eyewear for her various needs, LC laughs and says that she would lose her head if it were not attached. She is leery of having to keep track of multiple pairs of glasses and wants to try one pair to address all her needs. If you proceed with a multifocal, the distance prescription should be trial framed to probe for spatial distortion. If perception is altered and you reduce the amount of cylinder to minimize this effect, adjust the spherical equivalent to maintain the same net plus effect at near.

Looking at LC's distance findings, the subjective refraction is a spherical equivalent of –0.25 sph OU. If you reduce the cylinder by one diopter in each eye, the distance power to maintain the same spherical equivalent is

OD: Plano -0.50×75
OS: $+0.25 -1.00 \times 95$

To maintain the +3.00 spherical equivalent trial framed successfully for near, prescribe

OD: Plano $-0.50 \times 75 / + 3.25$
OS: $+0.25 -1.00 \times 95 / +3.25$

An argument could be made for tempering this prescription. In fact, it is a polite argument that LC might have when she returns with the following complaints:

- I am uncomfortable walking around with the glasses on.
- Watching television requires sitting upright.
- I have to search for the right spot.

Bear in mind that LC's original concern was related to reading for extended periods. Even though her over-the-counter readers did not incorporate cylinder, they give her a full field of view. She had over-the-counter readers stashed everywhere, and the pair in her nightstand were half-eyes so that she could glance at the TV comfortably. For the around-the-house purposes that LC envisions, consider moving more plus to the distance portion of the lens. This not only provides more useful power for television and other intermediate tasks but permits a reduction in add power, thereby reducing the distortion. Based on trial framing, you might arrive at the following power:

OD: $+0.75 -0.50 \times 75 / +2.50$
OS: $+1.00 -1.00 \times 95 / +2.50$

We close this chapter with the ultimate case of presbyopia, the pseudophakic patient. Although patients with IOLs (intraocular lenses) having undergone cataract surgery are discussed in Chapter 11, it is instructive to look at the case of an absolute presbyope who brings together in one case several of the rules we illustrate. See how well you can anticipate how we manage patient MV.

Subjective

Case History, Including Signs, Symptoms, and Visual Needs
Patient MV is a retired, 70-year-old patient with a history of high blood pressure and an irregular heart beat. His medication includes Coumadin ,which makes him susceptible to subconjunctival hemorrhages. He had been reluctant to have cataract surgery even though acuity in both eyes is steadily decreasing. The cataract in the left eye is more dense, and MV's distance acuity slowly dropped to 20/40 (6/12) OD and 20/70 (6/21) OS. He finally relents and is very pleased with his sight after having IOLs implanted in both eyes. MV jokes that when he tells friends he can now see the yellow lines on the road, they want to know why he did not warn them before. His eyes healed quickly after surgery, and he is ready for us to prescribe glasses. He has never had

a prescription for distance, and his previous reading glasses seem out of focus. MC is tall with long arms, and when we hand him a reading card he holds it reflexively at approximately 22 in. (56 cm) from his eyes.

Lensometry
OU: +3.00 –0.50 × 90 single vision for near only.

Objective

Ocular Health Assessment
Anterior chambers clear OU, pupils normal, IOLs clear and centered. IOP (intraocular pressure) is high normal in both eyes.

Clinical Measures

	At 20 ft (6 m)	At 16 in. (40 cm)
VA (unaided):	OD: 20/25 (6/7.5)	Deferred
	OS: 20/40 (6/12)	Deferred
Cover Test:	Ortho	Deferred
N.P.C.:	4 in./7 in. (10 cm/18 cm), limited by blur	
Retinoscopy/	OD: –0.25 sph	
Autorefractor:	OS: –0.75 –0.50 × 145	
Subjective:	OD: –0.25 sph	VA 20/20 (6/6)
	OS: –0.75 sph	VA 20/20 (6/6)
Phoria:	Ortho	5 exop
Base-in vergences:	N/E	X/16/12
Base-out vergences:	N/E	X/18/12

with near findings taken at 22 in. through +2.00 add

Accom. Amplitude:	Pseudophakia OU
Neg. Rel. Accom.:	Pseudophakia OU
Pos. Rel. Accom.:	Pseudophakia OU
Fused X-Cyl.:	+2.00 add, giving 20/20 (6/6) in each eye at 22 in. (56 cm)
Stereo:	30 seconds of arc

Assessment

MV is bilaterally pseudophakic with mild postsurgical myopic anisometropia.

Plan

1. Based on the near-point findings at MV's habitual reading distance, confirmed by trial framing, we gave MV a single vision prescription for near only with the following power:

   OD: +1.75

   OS: +1.25

   Note that, because MV is a myopic anisometrope, we factored the distance subjective into the selection of trial frame lenses for single vision at near. MV's habitual reading distance is 22 in. (56 cm), representing a dioptric demand of approximately 2.00 D over the distance subjective, resulting in a net power of +1.75 OD and +1.25 OS. A novice might mistakingly have the patient try to read through an equal power of +2.00 calculated for the near viewing distance demand, without taking into account the unequal plus lens factor induced by leaving the distance myopia uncorrected.

2. Another possibility is to prescribe a distance prescription in addition to the near prescription, or a multifocal prescription as follows:

   OD: −0.25/+2.00

   OS: −0.75/+2.00

   We would advise against this in MV's case for several reasons. He's a definitive person and indicated that he would rather not bother with a distance prescription. Trying to convince him otherwise would be unwise. Note the advantages that he has with his mild monovision effect when uncorrected. He actually will have an intermediate effect that will allow him to see his instrument panel better when driving and shelves when shopping or tooling around the house. His long arms give him a nice focal range with the −0.75 OS left uncorrected. MV has been used to driving with reduced acuity and contrast due to the cataracts for some time. With his IOLs, his overall vision is improved to the point that the residual low minus refraction is trivial compared to the way he was seeing before surgery. It would complicate his life keeping track of distance glasses, and multifocal glasses would require him to sacrifice the full field of view he enjoys with his single-vision lenses.

Consider another factor at this point. Would a distance prescription to achieve better binocular balance and stereopsis not be beneficial to MV for driving? Again, we advise against it. Patients with a cataract more advanced in one eye than the other have slowly decoupled their binocular sensitivity. By leaving MV's myopic anisometropia uncorrected at distance, you actually preserve the habitual dominance of the right eye for distance vision. The probability is that, if you prescribed distance glasses for MV, he would tell you that things are sharper but the prescription "doesn't feel right."

Tips on Multifocal Lensometry

As we demonstrated, the decisions a doctor makes about prescribing take the patient's habitual prescription into consideration. Three potential sources of error when an assistant or technician does lensometry on a presbyope's habitual prescription are common. When the patient has had her most recent examination in your office, the potential errors that we discuss can be avoided by comparing the lensometry finding to what was prescribed most recently.

Error 1

The technician asks the patient if she has glasses and, if so, what they are used for. The patient replies that she has reading glasses. The technician, presuming that the glasses are single vision for near only, neutralizes the glasses and comes up with +1.00 sph OU. The doctor does the examination, finds the optimal near power to be +1.75 sph OU, and demonstrates to the patient the large change that has occurred since her last prescription. The patient finds that odd since she perceives little change in ability to see clearly at near with her current glasses. The doctor looks at her glasses and realizes that she has a progressive lens. The power of the lenses is plano/+1.75 OU. The patient unintentionally misled the technician by telling him that she had reading glasses. This is understandable because the only time she puts the glasses on is to read. The technician, having no reason to think otherwise, simply centered the lens in the autolensometer and neutralized it halfway into the full power portion.

Error 2

The technician neutralizes a progressive addition lens prescription and registers the distance power at a point that already is into the corridor of the progressive. Therefore, relatively too much plus power is indicated for the distance portion and less plus power registers for the add value (Figure 6-5). Take a simple example:

Patient's actual prescription: OU: −1.00/+1.50
Prescription neutralized as: OU: −0.50/+1.00

In this case, the distance reads 0.50 less than it should because the measurement is incorrectly taken at a point +0.50 into the add, and the add therefore reads 0.50 less plus than it is. The net effect through the lens is still +0.50, but the relative values for distance and near are wrong.

Unless there is a previous prescription to check this against, detecting the error by looking at the lensometry printout is difficult. The doctor is more likely to discover this in a manner similar to error 1. When demonstrating the change in the distance prescription to the patient through the phoropter, the patient appreciates that the −1.00 sph OU is clearer than the −0.50 sph OU. But the patient may express surprise because she did not feel that her distance acuity had decreased. When the doctor has the patient put on her habitual glasses and she sees the chart clearly through them, the source of error in the neutralization becomes apparent.

An easier error to recognize is when the add powers differ between the two lenses, since unequal adds rarely are prescribed.

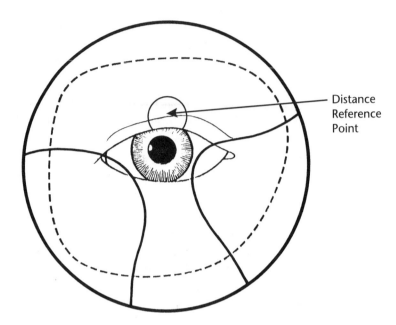

Figure 6-5 **Correct position of distance neutralization in progressive addition lens. The distance power in a progressive lens is verified at a higher point than in any other type of lens. The manufacturer supplies a semicircular mark for verification prior to dispensing. When neutralizing a patient's prescription as part of preliminary testing, this reference point is not available. Some autolensometers assist in locating this point, but if uncertain, always go to the upper region of the lens until the maximum minus or minimum plus portion is obtained.**

If the add in the right lens is not equal to the add in the left lens, assume that an error has been made in neutralizing the power until proven otherwise. Here is an example:

Patient's actual prescription: OU: –1.00/+1.50
Prescription neutralized as: OD: –1.00/+1.50
                                   OS: –0.50/+1.00

When the add power shows as unequal in the two eyes, the lens with the higher add power usually is correct. Therefore, the doctor would have the technician recheck the overall power in the left lens to see if the add power in fact is equal to the right lens.

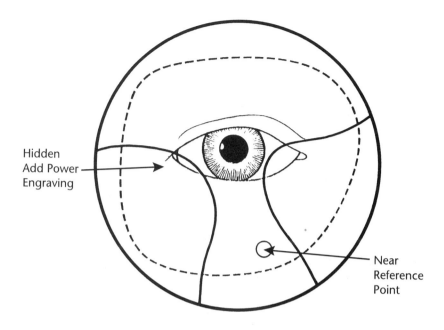

Hidden
Add Power
Engraving

Near
Reference
Point

Figure 6-6   Position of the progressive addition lens for maximum add power. Although progressive lenses have hidden add power engravings, they are not easily visible and usually not used by an assistant as part of the preliminary examination lens neutralization. When using the lensometer, look for the point of maximum add power toward the lowest nasal point on the lens where a reading can be obtained.

Error 3

A related error with progressive addition lenses is failure to get to the maximum add power. The maximum add value always is at the lowest portion of the lens and decentered nasally (Figure 6-6). In this instance, the distance portion of the prescription is located correctly, but less than the full add value is measured. When the technician fails to get to the proper location in both lenses, the shortfall on the add value will be similar in both eyes. For example,

Patient's actual prescription: OU: −1.00/+ 1.50
Prescription neutralized as: OU: −1.00/+1.00

In this instance, the doctor will have no clue that the neutralization is incorrect unless, as before, the patient's actual prescription is available. Particularly with a new patient, it would be easy for the doctor to conclude that the neutralized prescription is correct, and that the patient simply needs a significant increase in add power.

Error 4

This scenario is an error of omission rather than commission. The assistant neutralizes the lens prescription correctly, but the patient casually mentions that this is not her most recent prescription. The assistant fails to note this comment, and the doctor proceeds with the examination, thinking that the lensometry finding is what the patient is using habitually.

As demonstrated in this chapter, prescribing for presbyopia is an algorithmic reasoning process that is complete only when the doctor takes into account the diverse visual needs of adult patients.[20] Our general recommendations are summarized in Table 6-4. Prescribing successfully for presbyopic patients can be

---

Table 6-4   Synopsis of Pearls in Prescribing for Presbyopia

- Determine the patient's habitual working distance and prescribe at least one prescription maximizing clarity and range for the patient's most common working distance.
- Consider multiple prescriptions for specific vocational or avocational needs.
- Allow the patient to hold a magazine, newspaper, or representative work print in a comfortable position when trial framing.
- Select lens modalities that will not unduly compromise the functional visual field needed for work space.
- Measure the seg height with the patient's head in its natural position when looking straight ahead.
- If the patient has been happy with the habitual seg height, preserve the same relative seg height.
- Do not try to convince a patient who is happy with separate prescriptions for distance and near that he or she is unhappy.
- Do not try to convince a patient who is happy with a bifocal or trifocal that he or she has not lived until trying a progressive.

demanding at times, with all facets of optics coming into play. Early mistakes often are predictable and expensive, but the rewards that come with mastery are great.

References

1. Dunn S. *Different Hours.* New York: Norton, 2000:64–66.
2. Hofstetter HW, Griffin JR, Berman MS, Everson RW. *Dictionary of Visual Science and Related Clinical Terms*, 5th ed. Boston: Butterworth–Heinemann, 2000:407.
3. Kleinstein RN. Epidemiology of presbyopia. In: L Stark, G Obrecht (eds). *Presbyopia: Recent Research and Reviews from the Third International Symposium.* New York: Professional Press Books, 1987:12.
4. American Optometric Association. *Clinical Practice Guideline: Care of the Patient with Presbyopia.* St. Louis: American Optometric Association, 1998:4.
5. Grosvenor T. *Primary Care Optometry*, 4th ed. Boston: Butterworth–Heinemann, 2002:25.
6. Abrams D. *Duke-Elder's Practice of Refraction*, 10th ed. Edinburgh: Churchill Livingstone, 1993:92.
7. Kaufman PL. Accommodation and presbyopia: Neuromuscular and biophysical aspects. In: WM Hart (ed). *Adler's Physiology of the Eye.* St. Louis: Mosby/Year Book, 1992:391–411.
8. Milder B, Rubin ML. *The Fine Art of Prescribing Glasses without Making a Spectacle of Yourself*, 2nd ed. Gainesville, FL: Triad, 1991:102.
9. Rosenfield M, Ciuffreda KJ, Novogrodsky L. Contribution of accommodation and disparity vergence to transient near-work-induced myopic shifts. *Ophthal Physiol Opt.* 1992;12: 433–436.
10. Ong E, Ciuffreda KJ. *Accommodation, Nearwork and Myopia.* Santa Ana, CA: Optometric Extension Program, 1997:107.
11. Polasky M. Clinical refraction. In: KL Alexander (ed). *The Lippincott Manual of Primary Eye Care.* Philadelphia: Lippincott, 1995:190.
12. Birnbaum MH. *Optometric Management of Nearpoint Vision Disorders.* Boston: Butterworth–Heinemann, 1993:168.

13. Kurtz D. Presbyopia. In: KE Brookman (ed). *Refractive Management of Ametropia.* Boston: Butterworth–Heinemann, 1993: 154.

14. Holmes C, Joliffe H, Gregg J. *Guide to Occupational and Other Visual Needs.* Los Angeles: Silverlake Lithographers, 1958.

15. Sheedy JE. Vision problems at video display terminals: A survey of optometrists. *J Am Optom Assoc.* 1992;63:687–692

16. Anshel J. *Visual Ergonomics in the Workplace.* London: Taylor and Francis, 1998

17. Press LJ. Accommodative and vergence disorders: Restoring balance to a distressed system. In LJ Press (ed). *Applied Concepts in Vision Therapy.* St. Louis: Mosby, 1997.

18. Press LJ. Lenses and behavior. *J Optom Vis Devel.* 1990;21: 5–17.

19. Cho M. Case scenario 13. In: ER Ettinger, MW Rouse (eds). *Clinical Decision Making in Optometry.* Boston: Butterworth–Heinemann, 1997:318–327.

20. Ettinger ER. Clinical decision making skills. In: ER Ettinger, MW Rouse (eds). *Clinical Decision Making in Optometry.* Boston: Butterworth–Heinemann, 1997:4.

CHAPTER 7

Refractive Considerations in Binocular Vision Care

In presenting clinical perspectives on binocular vision at the primary care level, we limit ourselves to the commonplace and its contingencies. Clearly there is more. The subtitle of a book by David Koch on the 80/20 principle, "the secret of achieving more with less," could very well be the subtitle of this chapter.[1]

> 80/20 Thinking is my phrase for the applications of the 80/20 Principle to daily life, for nonquantitative applications of the principle. As with 80/20 Analysis, we start with a hypothesis about a possible imbalance between inputs and outputs, but, instead of collecting data and analyzing them, we estimate them. 80/20 Thinking requires, and with practice enables, us to spot the few really important things that are happening and ignore the mass of unimportant things. It teaches us to see the wood for the trees. 80/20 Thinking is too valuable to be confined to causes where data and analysis are perfect. For every ounce of insight generated quantitatively, there must be pounds of insight arrived at intuitively and impressionistically. This is why 80/20 Thinking, although helped by data, must not be constrained by it.

We hope not to offend anyone with the following statement, but it is central to the premise of this chapter. Most optometrists will find that 80% of binocular anomalies can be managed effectively with 20% of the data they were taught in courses on binocular vision and physiological optics. As with our approach to other clinical matters, it is not meant to suggest that there are no alternative approaches. Most sources that address binocular vision problems place a heavy emphasis on AC/A, CA/C, fixation disparity, classification of syndromes, hypothetical etiologies, vision therapy, and so forth. While we acknowledge that such considerations are important for select patients and a source of interest for a select number of practitioners, it simply is not the way refractive decisions are made by the strong majority of our profession. Some cases warrant detailed analysis while others can be managed effectively without detailed analysis or theory.

Isometropic Changes in Prescription

Changes in isometropic lens prescriptions, particularly when differing less than 1 diopter from the habitual state, rarely induce binocular dysfunction. In most cases, the patient's symptoms can be attributed to changes in spatial perception, and the patient adapts uneventfully. However, **clinical pearl 8** advises that it often is prudent in making a lens change of more than 1 diopter to prescribe it in stages. In addition to having to adapt to spatial changes at distance, the patient may encounter adjustments in binocular vision at near point. Patients with a high-gradient AC/A experience an initial shift in phoria when the lens power changes.

It has become popular within optometry to use John Potter's designation of the optimal endpoint acuity as 20/Happy. This certainly is the case when moderating lens prescriptions to achieve the best balance between visual acuity and binocular function and comfort. Changes in lens prescription become more significant when the patient is marginally compensating for a binocular imbalance through the habitual lens prescription. This is particularly true when the patient has esophoria and progressive myopia. Consider the following example of a 16 year old with complaints of distance blur:

Lensometry:	–2.00 sphere OU
Habitual DVA:	20/60 (6/18) OD/OS
Habitual Phoria:	Distance = ortho
Subjective Refraction:	–3.00 sphere OU
Phoria Through –3.00:	Distance = 8 eso

NFV Through −3.00:	Distance BI = X/4/2
Gradient AC/A:	−1.00/ 8$^\Delta$

At first glance it looks like the patient will have trouble adjusting to the extra −1.00 D, because she has a narrow margin to diplopia. This is the patient we discussed in Chapter 3 who would report, if trial framed, that things look sharper at distance, but that the full power makes her eyes feel strange. This is why **clinical pearl 8** advises trial framing the tentative increase in lens power if it is more than 1 diopter.

If we make a lens change that requires significant binocular adaptation, we could hope for the best and encourage the patient that she will adapt successfully. If we are to recheck the successfully adapted patient in 2 weeks, we likely would find that the distance phoria has lessened or that the negative fusional vergence (base-in) range at distance has increased. However, another possibility is to prescribe less of an increase in the lens prescription at the outset. Increasing the power to −2.50 instead of −3.25 still provides a significant increase in acuity from the habitual state. This would lessen the esophoria at the outset and enable the patient to operate more within a fusional zone of comfort.

When tempering the distance prescription, deciding on the amount of power to lessen or add in aiding the binocular vision profile may be done empirically.[2] Criteria that can be used to select the tentative lens for trial framing can be a power that enables the patient to satisfy Morgan's or Optometric Extension Program norms, Sheard's criterion, or puts the patient more in line with a desirable fixation disparity profile. With clinical experience, practitioners find it equally effective to use a lens flipper demonstrator of +/−0.50 and +/−1.00, hold it over the patient's current glasses while he or she looks out the window, and ask about subjective changes in both clarity and comfort.

Anisometropia for the Ages

Anisometropia, a difference in power between the two eyes in either or both of the principal meridians, becomes clinically significant in the amount of 1 diopter or more.[3] The lens prescription for a patient with anisometropia varies, depending on the amount of anisometropia, the age of the patient, and the patient's binocular status. Although we do not emphasize a behavioral approach to lenses in this discussion, interested readers are encouraged to consult compendia representative of alternative approaches to lens prescribing.[4,5]

Polasky summarizes traditional insights into anisometropia, providing a cornucopia of clinical pearls.[6] We have taken the liberty of elaborating on them as follows:

1. *Uncorrected anisometropia rarely results in awareness of blur with both eyes open.* Depending on the distance the patient is viewing, the brain simply taps into the eye with better acuity. This is true when anisometropia has been present for a significant period of time or evolved slowly. When anisometropia is acquired rapidly (for example, when a side effect of a drug or disease), the adult patient may be aware of blur in one or both eyes or, in rare instances, diplopia.

2. *Small amounts of uncorrected anisometropia tend to cause more symptoms than larger amounts of anisometropia. When anisometropia exceeds 1 diopter, the patient tends to view with one eye and suppresses the other eye.* The suppression process in these cases may be detected clinically by using small targets showing central suppression or by testing stereopsis. Examination with a vectographic slide usually reveals suppression when measuring distance visual acuities. The patient is likely to remain asymptomatic when left uncorrected.

3. *Since suppression often accompanies uncorrected anisometropia, amblyopia is a distinct possibility. Amblyopia is more likely with uncorrected anisometropic hyperopia than with anisometropic myopia. In anisometropic hyperopia, the eye requiring less accommodation to see clearly is the preferred eye. The other eye is likely to be suppressed, leading to functional amblyopia.* Uncompensated myopic anisometropia under 4 diopters rarely results in amblyopia because the patient uses the less myopic eye for distance and the more myopic eye for near, maintaining good visual acuity in both eyes. When anisometropia exceeds 4 diopters, the patient is not likely to adjust the near working

distance to keep the more myopic eye conjugate. Uncompensated hyperopic anisometropia above 2 diopters, and occasionally of lesser value, often results in amblyopia of the eye with greater hyperopia. Being economical, the visual system tends to accommodate only the amount needed to clear the image through the less hyperopic eye, leaving the more hyperopic eye blurred at distance and near. Even when treated with patching in conjunction with prescription lenses, patients with hyperopic anisometropia greater than 1.50 diopters are at risk for the amblyopia recurring after occlusion therapy is stopped, and they must be closely monitored.[7] The effects of uncompensated astigmatism on visual acuity vary depending on the resultant spherical equivalent as well as the orientation of the cylinder axes, with uncompensated oblique axes being more amblyogenic. The amblyopia induced by uncorrected astigmatism, known as *meridional refractive amblyopia*, is discussed in Chapter 5. General guidelines for lens prescribing to minimize the development of anisometropic amblyopia are given in Table 7-1.

4. *In certain cases, the correction of anisometropia will lead to symptoms of headache, asthenopia, and visual distortion. This usually is prism induced when patients view objects through the peripheral portion of their spectacle lenses. In the case examples later in*

Table 7-1   Guidelines to Minimize Anisometropic Amblyopia

Refractive Status	*Risk Factor*	*Suggested Prescription*
Myopia	Above 4 D	Full prescription with contact lenses when possible. If natural monovision, undercorrect to maintain more myopic eye for near.
Hyperopia	Above 1 D	Minimize aniso and prescribe conservatively. Refraction tends to be labile; recheck frequently during sensitive periods.
Astigmatism	Above 1 D	Not labile after age 2. Prescribe fully if repeatable. Be more aggressive in childhood when cylinder axes are oblique.
Antimetropia	Above 1 D	Follow same suggestions as for myopia and hyperopia.

this chapter, we place considerable emphasis on the trade-off between maximum visual acuity and maximum visual comfort and function. Many patients with robust vertical prism adaptation have little or no difficulty accepting significant anisometropic lens prescriptions.[8,9] Although prism induced when looking away from the optical centers can be problematic with single-vision lenses, it is a greater source of difficulty in multifocal lens form, and can be compensated for with a slab-off prism design. A patient who has symptoms of visual discomfort relieved by occluding one eye and no vergence or accommodative problem would be better served by having a separate pair of single-vision spectacles for near use.

5. *When a slab-off prism is required to enable comfortable use of multifocals, the following guidelines are useful:*

   • Measure the amount of induced vertical prism with a Maddox rod while the patient looks at a light in the normal reading position through the net near lens values that will be prescribed. It is most convenient to use a Maddox rod with a built-in Risley prism (available from Bernell Corporation). Another way to measure vertical imbalance directly is to use the associated vertical phoria value. This is the amount of prism necessary to level the nonius lines on a vertical fixation disparity measurement.

   • The amount of slab-off prism measured or prescribed often is less than what is calculated based on Prentice's rule for the amount of vertical imbalance induced by anisometropia in the vertical meridian. As with all cases of vertical prism, it is better to stay on the conservative side.

   • Stock flat-top segments are available in powers ranging from 1.5 to 6 prism diopters, and labs such as Vision-Ease are helpful with reverse slab-off and custom orders.[10]

   • Slab-off prism is cosmetically noticeable and produces significant image jump at the junction line. It is least noticeable when the slab-off line is coincident with a flat-top line and the minimum amount of slab off is required (1.5 prism diopters).

6. *Aniseikonia is induced in certain cases by anisometropic lens prescriptions.* Prescribe contact lenses for anisometropia whenever possible. Even when aniseikonia is predicted to be significant with contact lenses due to Knapp's law of axial versus refractive image size differences, attempt a contact lens correction. In our clinical experience, the induced prism through spectacle lenses, and the resultant anisophoria in different directions of gaze, nearly always is more of a problem than image size differences. As with other types of binocular imbalance, it is easier to adapt to constant errors such as aniseikonia than the variable imbalances induced by anisophoria. There are other points of view on this subject.[11–13]

Lens Additions and Binocular Dysfunction

Most optometric practitioners agree that the influence of a lens prescription on binocular vision occurs principally through a dual interactive model of vergence accommodation, involving AC/A and CA/C crossover effects. Prescription lenses for ametropia, even of small magnitude, can dramatically improve vergence and accommodative function for many patients.[14] There are other schools of thought, and again we refer the interested reader to alternative considerations regarding the effect of lenses on binocular vision.[15] We intersperse some behavioral observations to supplement and, in some cases, supplant traditional thinking. We now look at three conditions where a lens prescription or addition has a direct impact on binocular function. Specifically, we consider accommodative esotropia, pseudoconvergence insufficiency, and divergence excess.

Accommodative Esotropia

The most widespread application of lenses to influence binocular vision is the case of plus lenses to reduce accommodative esotropia. When the AC/A ratio is high, a relatively low amount of plus has a significant effect on lessening overconvergence. For clinical purposes, it is valid to use the gradient method to calculate AC/A.[16] As an example, if an emmetropic patient measures 14 prism diopters of esophoria at near with no lenses in place and the angle reduces to 10 prism diopters of esophoria when remeasured through +1.00, the gradient AC/A is 4/1.

The clinical aim of prescribing a plus lens addition in accommodative esotropia is to convert the tropia to a phoria. Naturally, the plus lens prescription can be coupled with any other intervention that enhances binocular vision such as base-out prism, binasal occlusion, or other forms of vision therapy. If the plus lens power that lessens the eso at near will not be accepted at distance, it is prescribed in multifocal lens form. As noted in **clinical pearl 7**, when esophoria at distance causes problems or it is difficult to prescribe an add, the practitioner may cautiously push a little more plus lens power at distance if the patient tolerates a modest reduction in visual acuity. This is particularly true when cycloplegia or delayed subjective manifest refraction confirms the existence of latent hyperopia. If the patient is a child, the practitioner should recheck the prescription frequently to confirm the optimal amount of plus lens power at distance and near that balances acuity, alignment, comfort, posture, and performance.

Rosner and Rosner present the application of lenses through case examples of hyperopia associated with intermittent esotropia of the convergence excess type, as well as constant esotropia secondary to significant hyperopia.[17] A key component in managing cases of this nature is to monitor the child's progress. Multifocals prescribed to control overconvergence when the child is younger may be switched to single-vision lenses as the child grows older. In all cases, it is important to prepare the child's parents for the probability that one eye or the other will continue to visibly turn inward when the glasses are removed.

We wish we had the space to quote Caloroso and Rouse's discussion of lens application.[18] Among the many pearls in the chapter on lens therapy is the reminder that patients with significant hyperopia still require a lens prescription after their eyes are surgically aligned. As they note, apparent straightness of eye position is not equivalent to visual efficiency or even binocular vision. Wearing the appropriate lens prescription (as deduced by methods for determining plus lens acceptance) preserves visual efficiency. Dismissing the need for lenses after surgery is one reason why some children reestablish strabismus after being apparently aligned.

Pseudoconvergence Insufficiency

Originally termed *false convergence insufficiency*, pseudoconvergence insufficiency is a condition resulting in a remote near point of convergence secondary to a reduced accommodative response. Anything that can be done to improve accommodative responses also improves the convergence.[19] Although not included in the classical binocular syndromes described by Duane and White, pseudoconvergence insufficiency is not uncommon in optometric practice.[20] Richman and Cron observed that a plus lens add can improve the near point of convergence in cases of pseudoconvergence insufficiency.[21]

At first blush, it may seem surprising that an add can improve convergence insufficiency. This result would seem to go against the grain of what is predicted by graphical analysis. Plus lenses theoretically should induce more exophoria. The explanation given for this paradox is that the condition is primarily an accommodative insufficiency, supported by a high lag of accommodation noted on crossed cylinder testing or near-point retinoscopy. Given some help in accommodating, the patient can reactivate at least some of the accommodation that was lagging. This in turn helps to pull in accommodative convergence, thereby lessening the secondary underconvergence.[16] In their discussion of pseudoconvergence insufficiency, Scheiman and Wick report a case where low plus lenses for near did not initially improve the near point of convergence but nonetheless were prescribed and proved beneficial in conjunction with vision therapy.[11]

We emphasize this topic because it highlights the importance of discarding a traditional model of accommodation and convergence in those instances where it does not fit for specific patients. It seems more plausible in cases of this nature to assume that these patients engage in functional inhibition to reduce near-point stress-induced overcongergence.[22] This is another way of saying that at least some of the patients with convergence insufficiency originally were esophoric and adapted by underaccommodating or underconverging. The decision to try added lenses and observe the effect on their binocular vision should not be constrained by calculated AC/A ratios or case type labels. In other words, what harm can be done by taking a pair of +0.50 lenses out of the trial case, holding them in front of the patient, and seeing what the subjective response is? You might reinforce this by using a lens demonstrator with a pair of +0.50 lenses on one side and –0.50 lenses on the other side, to see if the patient can differentiate between the feeling or comfort of looking through one set of lenses versus the other.

The majority of convergence insufficiencies are of the true rather than pseudo type, and added plus lenses at near increases the exophoria. Although induced high exophoria and convergence insufficiency with added plus lenses at near can occur at any age, it can be an overlooked source of difficulty in reading in presbyopia. We tend to attribute near-point complaints in presbyopia solely to loss of accommodation or, half-jokingly, to the general fatigue associated with aging. Convergence insufficiency always should be considered a potential cause of near-point symptomatology at any age and lenses, prisms, or vision therapy presented as treatment options when indicated. When the add value and AC/A are high, base-in prism usually is needed to offset the increased exophoria induced by the plus lenses.[23]

Intermittent Exotropia at Distance (Divergence Excess)

When the patient has high exophoria or intermittent exotropia at distance, can added minus lenses at distance be used effectively to stimulate convergence? Yes, theoretically, as long as the patient has a relatively high-gradient AC/A and an adequate accommodative amplitude to absorb the excessive accommodation at distance without experiencing asthenopia. How much added minus lens power theoretically would it take to attain alignment at distance? The lens power is calculated by first determining the

AC/A ratio, then determining the lens value that reduces the exotropia by the desired amount.

$$AC/A = PD \text{ (cm)} + \frac{\text{near deviation} - \text{far deviation}}{\text{near focus} - \text{far focus}}$$

In this formula, the deviation is in prism diopters with exo taking a minus value and eso taking a plus value. Look at an example suggested by Grisham.[2]

A 12-year-old child has an intermittent exotropia at distance of 18 prism diopters and a near exophoria of 8 prism diopters at 40 cm. The PD is 60 mm. According to the preceding formula:

$$AC/A = 6 + \frac{-8 - (-18)}{2.5 - 0}$$

Therefore, with an AC/A of 10/1, the amount of lens power to reduce the 18 prism diopter exotropia to 0 would be −1.75. However, it is always preferable to prescribe the least amount of added power needed. Therefore, it may be more practical to simply add −1.00 sph OU, redo the cover test, and note the effect. It is possible in cases with a high-gradient AC/A that lesser added lens values will pull in the patient enough to convert the intermittent tropia to a phoria.

If the added minus lenses cause asthenopia, particularly when secondary near-point problems are induced, a near add can be prescribed to offset the added minus at distance.[24] We might think that prescribing lenses to encourage overaccommodation at distance would be a trigger to the development of myopia. Studies to date have not borne this out.[25] However, high exophoria or intermittent exotropia at distance may be resistant to the added lens approach because the response AC/A ratio is not as high as is commonly suggested. Coupled with the observation that fusional vergence ranges in this condition typically are normal, this calls into question the ability of clinicians to successfully manage divergence excess simply as a problem of high phoria.[11] The point here is to be careful about managing high exophoria or intermittent exotropia at distance with added minus lenses in the absence of vision therapy. At the very least, we have to be prepared to prescribe an add and monitor the patient closely.

Prism and Binocular Dysfunction

Prescribing prism for binocular dysfunction is an underutilized option. One strong reason for this is the blanket and unwarranted fear many clinicians have about patients requiring increasing amounts of prism once the first prism power has been prescribed. Cotter addresses this perception in the Preface to her compilation on the clinical applications of prism.[26] On the flip side, vergence adaptation can be troublesome for clinicians who are cavalier about prescribing prism for binocular dysfunction. Patients with robust, slow vergence systems readily adapt to prescribed prism and are better managed through vision therapy.[27]

In the pursuit of binocular Nirvana, we tend to follow clinical guidelines for prescribing prism similar to the unifying concepts suggested by Saladin.[28] As Saladin notes, comfort criteria such as Percival's and Sheard's were not based on statistical evidence but intuitive beliefs that any system should have a certain position or reserve within the continuum of its range. It differs little from a conservative investor suggesting we keep a third of our funds in reserve for demanding financial times. Percival's criterion has not withheld scrutiny in regard to binocular comfort, but Sheard's criterion has stood the test of time and is particularly useful for patients with exophoria.

Sheard postulated that, for any given fixation distance, the reserve of the compensating ranges should be at least equal to twice the demand of the phoria. The blur finding is used as the reserve value. In the absence of a blur finding, the break represents the reserve value. We take as an example a patient with 9 exophoria at near. The blur or break value should be at least 18 prism diopters. To determine the amount of prism to prescribe if the break value is less than 18 prism diopters, use the following formula:

$$P = \tfrac{2}{3}D - \tfrac{1}{3}R$$

For our symptomatic patient with 9 exophoria at near and a break of only 12 prism diopters, the amount of base-in prism indicated at near is

$$P = \tfrac{2}{3}(9) - \tfrac{1}{3}(12) = 2 \text{ prism diopters}$$

For patients with esophoria, prescribing prism to meet Sheard's criterion is not as reliable. Rather than using the break value as with Sheard's, Saladin suggests using the recovery as the reserve value. The base-in recovery should be at least equal to the phoria. This is known as the *1:1 criterion*. To determine the amount of base-out prism to prescribe for esophoria, use the following formula:

$$P = (D - R)/2$$

Consider a symptomatic patient with 6 prism diopters of esophoria at near and a base-in recovery value of 2 prism diopters. Since the recovery is less than 6 prism diopters, the 1:1 criterion is not met and the amount of base-out prism to be prescribed is calculated as

$$P = (6 - 2)/2 = 2 \text{ prism diopters}$$

For esophoria at near, plus lenses may be used at near to substitute for the calculated base-out prism value, in accordance with the formula $S = P/A$. In this formula, S is the spherical lens value, P is the calculated prism, and A is the AC/A ratio. For expediency, the gradient AC/A usually is used. Taking the preceding example, we remeasure the near phoria at 40 cm through a +1.00 lens and find that the 6 esophoria reduces to 2 esophoria.. The gradient AC/A is 4/1. To determine the lens value to substitute for the base-out prism calculated by the 1:1 criterion,

$$S = P/A$$
$$S = 2/4 = +0.50$$

Vertical phorias present a different challenge. Even small amounts of vertical prism, particularly those that persist after compensation of lateral phorias, can cause significant symptoms.

The most common approach to prescribing prism for vertical imbalances is to prescribe the amount of the associated phoria as determined during fixation disparity testing. This is the amount of vertical prism required to reduce fixation disparity to 0.[29] As cited by Goss, an earlier approach suggested by Borish uses the amount of prism that balances the vertical fusion amplitudes as follows:

$$P = \frac{(\text{base down to break}) - (\text{base up to break})}{2}$$

A positive P value indicates a base-down prism and a negative P value indicates a base-up prism. For example, a patient with 2 right hyperphoria measures a base-down break of 6 and a base-up break of 3. According to the formula,

$$P = \frac{(6) - (3)}{2} = 1.5$$

The patient is prescribed 1.5 prism diopters base down in front of the right eye. Prism usually is split between the two eyes, unless fixation disparity shows the principal drift to be referenced more to one eye than the other. Vision therapy to alter vertical vergence ranges, although more difficult to achieve than expanding lateral ranges, may be undertaken to limit the amount of vertical prism necessary.[30] As a general rule, it always is preferable to prescribe the minimum amount of prism necessary to reduce symptoms or enhance performance.

In summary, the following are general guidelines adapted from Saladin:[28]

Convergence Insufficiency: First try vision therapy and, if the symptoms persist, prescribe prism to meet Sheard's criterion.

Convergence Excess: Try plus lenses at near first, then vision therapy or base-out prism as needed.

Divergence Excess: First try vision therapy. Prism may be used with therapy, according to the

	discussion in the section on intermittent exotropia at distance.
Divergence Insufficiency:	Prescribe base-out prism to meet the 1:1 criterion at distance. The same amount of prism usually is acceptable at near.
Basic Exophoria:	Prescribe base-in prism to meet Sheard's criterion. If latent exophoria exists, implement vision therapy.
Basic Esophoria:	Prescribe base-out prism to meet the 1:1 criterion. If symptoms persist, prescribe prism to put the operating point on the flat portion of the fixation disparity curve.
Vertical Phoria:	Prescribe the associated phoria value if symptomatic.

The effects of prism addressed are limited to traditional prescribing for vergence dysfunction. Other sources may be consulted for the effects of prism on spatial localization and general behavioral function.[4,31]

Induced Prismatic Changes

Clinical pearl 12, advising caution in changing the lens design with high prescriptions, warrants further discussion here. An interesting conundrum arises when the patient has induced prism in the habitual lens prescription. This might have occurred because of unintended decentration effects. Take, for example, the patient who says that he went back to the doctor who prescribed the glasses 2 years ago, having had the sensation that something was wrong with the prescription. The doctor checked the lens power, determined that it was correct, and advised him that it would take a little time to adapt to the new eyewear. After examining the patient, you find no indication for prism, but the patient has adapted to the unintended horizontal or vertical prism present in the lenses. If you remove the prism, the patient theoretically will have to adapt again. Our clinical experience has been that, in most cases, the prism can be removed without disturbing the patient when it is present in small amounts. However, whenever a sensitive patient has trouble adjusting to a new prescription, compare the comfortable eyewear to the new eyewear to determine if the comfortable prescription induced prism. If so, duplicate the same prism power in the new eyewear. The decision need not be absolute. If the prism is of an appreciable amount it can be cut in half.

Although it has been demonstrated that Prentice's rule is an oversimplification,[32] we use it to illustrate the point of unintended prism. A 30-year-old patient with a 54 mm PD and a prescription of –5.00 sph OU reports being comfortable with her current glasses. You examine her, determine that her power has remained the same, and therefore reissue the prescription for –5.00 sph OU at her anatomical PD (APD) of 54 mm. After selecting new eyewear and receiving her glasses, she complains of trouble adjusting to the new glasses. She now remembers that the same thing happened with her previous eyewear, and it took several months before she felt comfortable with the lenses. You take a closer look at the previous eyewear and note that the mechanical PD (MPD) is actually at 64 mm. In accordance with Prentice's rule,

$$\text{MPD (cm)} - \text{APD (cm)} \times \text{power} = \text{Induced prism}$$
$$(6.4 - 5.4) \times (5) = 5 \text{ prism diopters}$$

Since it is a minus lens prescription and the lenses have been effectively decentered outward from the APD, the resultant prism is in the base-in direction. This would tend to make the patient more uncomfortable if she is esophoric, particularly if she has poor negative fusional vergence (base-in) ranges. But she has adapted to the lenses. Now if we remake the lenses at the actual APD of 54 mm, we introduce a change of 5 prism diopters in the base-out direction compared to the habitual eyewear. If the patient has adequate fusional convergence (base-out) ranges, this may not be an issue.

Bear in mind that, as reviewed in Chapter 3 on myopia, one way to keep the edge thickness of minus lenses to a minimum is to minimize lens decentration. So it is entirely possible that **clinical pearl 15** is in effect here: The patient's last eye doctor may have been wiser than you initially thought. The outward decentration of the patient's lenses from her APD was no error but a purposeful change to put the MPD close to a 0 decentration value for cosmetic purposes. The previous practitioner may have even taken the patient's overall binocular status into consideration. The doctor also may have thought it was simpler telling the patient that she would get used to the new eyewear than go through an optical explanation of why the MPD did not match the APD, as it had in her previous eyewear.

In summary, we have several options in this case:

1. Fill the new prescription at the habitual PD if the patient is asymptomatic. This is the guideline offered in **clinical pearl 12**.
2. Fill the new prescription at the APD. This would be advisable if the patient has convergence excess and avoided the symptoms of poorly compensated esophoria by reading less. A return to the APD should help.
3. If the patient reports difficulty adapting to the new lenses, shift the lens PD midway between the habitual MPD and the patient's APD.

Binocular Adaptation Following Refractive Surgery

Whenever the optical correction is moved posteriorly from the spectacle plane, a binocular adaptation is required. In myopia, the demand on accommodation and convergence increases when switching from the spectacle plane to the corneal plane.[33] The esophoric myope is at greatest risk for experiencing symptoms of near-point discomfort when switching from spectacles to contact lenses.[34] Greater amounts of adaptation are required as the power of the spectacle lens prescription increases.

Although not as widely recognized, a similar adaptation is required in pseudophakia, when the correcting plane switches from spectacle lenses to intraocular lenses (IOLs). In most cases, both the patient's eyes are not operated on at the same time. This leaves the patient with a period of induced anisometropia, which may not be as significant a problem as we would anticipate. In most cases, binocularity has been compromised to some extent for a period of time, as lens changes occur asymmetrically. As the acuity diminishes in one eye more than the other eye, a suppression process builds to avoid diplopia. We touched on this in the last chapter, in the case of patient MV.

In cases of unilateral pseudophakia, when the fellow eye has no significant lenticular opacification, the surgeon may calculate the implant power to match the ametropia of the fellow eye and minimize anisometropia. If the fellow eye subsequently requires an IOL, the surgeon then uses an implant power to match the IOL to the first IOL. In a small percentage of cases, patients with pseudophakia will experience diplopia and require prism or vision therapy to assist with fusion. If neither approach is feasible, fogging one eye or occlusion may be necessary.

Less recognized are the implications for difficulties in binocular adaptation after corneal refractive surgery.[35] Accommodative and binocular findings in previously normal patients may be altered and can induce asthenopia in some subjects that persists as long as 18 months after the procedure.[36] In other instances, a patient with fragile binocularity prior to refractive surgery may emerge from the procedure with adequate visual clarity but decompensated binocular function.[37] We raise these issues because, as refractive surgery becomes more commonplace, some segment of this population will have asthenopic complaints that may be attributed to dry eyes or residual, uncompensated refractive power. However, in a subset of patients, the accommodative or binocular status after surgery contributes to symptomology. This will be more of a challenge for those patients who have refractive surgery without having had the prior experience of contact lenses and therefore must make a sudden shift in correction from the spectacle plane to the corneal plane.

Undoubtedly, dry eye syndrome and other factors contributing to visual fatigue such as glare must be taken into account when the patient has lingering symptoms after refractive surgery. However, accommodative and binocular findings should be checked to see if the patient's function can be improved through added lenses, prism, or vision therapy.

Case Examples

Subjective

Case History, Including Signs, Symptoms, and Visual Needs

BB, a 44-year-old publishing assistant, does a lot of computer work. Last year, we gave her prescription lenses, primarily for use when driving or engaged in other distance activities. When she returns for her examination this year, she tells us sheepishly that she rarely uses the glasses. Although she noticed that things are clearer when she wears the glasses, it takes so long to readjust her focus after taking them off that it just was not worth it. In her words, it was like a shock to her system.

Lensometry
OD: $-1.00 -0.25 \times 40$
OS: Plano -0.50×110

Objective

Ocular Health Assessment
All findings normal.

Clinical Measures

	At 20 ft (6 m)	At 16 in. (40 cm)
VA (unaided):	OD: 20/50 (6/15)	20/20 (6/6)
	OS: 20/50 (6/15)	20/20 (6/6)
Cover Test:	Ortho	Sl exo
N.P.C.:	N/E	
Retinoscopy/	OD: $-1.75 -0.25 \times 46$	
Autorefractor:	OS: $+0.25 -1.00 \times 115$	
Subjective:	OD: $-1.00 -0.25 \times 40$	VA 20/20 (6/6)
	OS: $+0.25 -0.50 \times 110$	VA 20/20 (6/6)
Phoria:	Ortho	Sl exo
Base-in vergences:	N/E	N/E
Base-out vergences:	N/E	N/E

Accom. Amplitude:	N/E
Neg. Rel. Accom.:	N/E
Pos. Rel. Accom.:	N/E
Fused X-Cyl.:	N/E
Stereo:	N/E

Assessment

Early presbyopia with anisometropia.

Plan

We reassure BB that, if she feels more comfortable in general by not wearing glasses, she should hold them in reserve for the future. No harm would be done by not wearing the lenses, and the changes that would occur in the future are not influenced by the decision to limit use of the prescription. In reviewing BB's record, it was evident that she has natural monovision, preferring the right eye for near and intermediate and the left eye for distance. The only reason we decide to give her a distance prescription is because each year we ask if she feels like there are any changes with her vision. Last year, for the first time, she acknowledged that, when driving in unfamiliar places at night, she could not detect signs as quickly as she had in the past.

Much of the potentially collectable binocular findings do not contribute to the decision-making process in this case. As indicated elsewhere, it is certainly noble to take these findings to round out the data. But, if there are time constraints, either on the part of the practitioner or the patient, the time is better spent discussing the potential benefits versus trade-offs that occur in prescribing lenses or recommending any other form of intervention. The key to this case is that BB basically is asymptomatic, and attempts to compensate for the myopia of the right eye with a lens prescription creates a problem by attempting to enhance binocular vision. In essence, we have a corollary of **clinical pearl 3**, which indicates that every myope has a right to her seeing preferences. BB prefers not having her myopia compensated for because that forces her into a binocular viewing situation that is uncomfortable and deprives her of the monovision effect, which provides a full range of focus without lenses.

Bear in mind that a patient having natural monovision has acquired this condition slowly, differentiating it from doctor-induced monovision. The adaptation required in this case would be to the doctor's suggestion that more balanced binocular vision at distance is an ideal worth pursuing. Say, hypothetically, that BB were to have come in for her appointment this year telling us that she was unable to wear the prescription comfortably and distance blur when driving at night still is an issue. Even though we trial framed the prescription last year to acceptance in the office, there is room to compromise so that we preserve some of BB's mono-vision effect. Consider that, when she is driving at night, BB relies on her right eye for peripheral awareness, and her left eye for central detail. It is difficult to simulate this dynamic situation in the static confines of the office. Therefore, instead of the prescription we gave her last year, we could preserve more of her habitual balance between the two eyes by reducing her prescription to

OD: –0.50 sphere
OS: Plano –0.50 × 110

This is where some of the art overlaps the science. We have speculated that some of BB's sensation of a "shock to her system" when she put on the glasses is due to the asymmetrical oblique astigmatism. The partial prescription would reduce that effect.

Consider another alternative in prescribing. In looking back on BB's record, we note that her right eye has remained stable in the amount of myopia, but the left eye cylindrical power has surfaced in only the past 2 years. We might then assume that, since BB relies on her left eye for distance detail, we should be refining the left eye for distance and the right eye should remain uncorrected. We therefore propose giving BB the following prescription:

OD: Plano
OS: +0.25 –0.50 × 110

All these options could be confusing, so we take a clear stand. If BB asks whether we can modify her glasses to make things more comfortable when she uses them for night driving, we hold a +0.50 sph trial lens in front of her current right lens. We do this under low-light conditions, looking at signage in the office or out the window. We wait for her to report feeling more comfortable, while remaining sharper than when she removes the prescription eyewear. If so, we go with the reduced myopic prescription. If she finds it improved but still feels strange, we remove the lens from the right eye and have BB repeat the test with only the left eye having a prescription lens in place.

Last, we point out that vision therapy might be a consideration in BB's case. However, we must weigh the cost/benefit ratio of opening up a Pandora's box of sorts in these situations, particularly in adulthood. If BB has specific symptoms that would benefit from vision therapy beyond the occasional use of a distance prescription, vision therapy would be compelling.

Subjective

Case History, Including Signs, Symptoms, and Visual Needs
DL is a 9-year-old child who has bifocals prescribed by another doctor. She reports doing well in school but complains of distance blur lately. The glasses do not seem to help, and she has been using them only periodically for reading. Her general health is normal, and she takes no medications.

Lensometry
OU: Plano/+2.50

Objective

Ocular Health Assessment
All findings normal.

Clinical Measures

	At 20 ft (6 m)	At 16 in. (40 cm)
VA (unaided):	OD: 20/60 (6/18)	20/20 (6/6)
	OS: 20/50 (6/15)	20/20 (6/6)

	At 20 ft (6 m)	*At 16 in. (40 cm)*
Cover Test:	Ortho	Alt E(T)'
N.P.C.:	To the nose	
Retinoscopy/	OD: –1.50 sphere	
Autorefractor:	OS: –1.25 sphere	
Subjective:	OD: –1.50 sphere	VA 20/20
	OS: –1.25 sphere	VA 20/20
Phoria:	8 eso	Alt E(T)'
Base-in vergences:	X/2/–6	Suppr
Base-out vergences:	X/20/16	Suppr
Accom. Amplitude:	10 diopters	
Neg. Rel. Accom.:	Suppr	
Pos. Rel. Accom.:	Suppr	
Fused X-Cyl.:	Suppr	
Stereo:	Suppr	

Assessment

Low myopia with accommodative esotropia.

Plan

We gave DL the following prescription: –0.50 sph OU/+2.50.

DL's chief complaint is blurred distance vision. When we trial frame the distance subjective refraction, DL reports sharper vision but notices ghost imaging, which turns out to be intermittent diplopia. This fragile fusion is not surprising based on her esophoria at distance and tenuous base in vergence range. At near, DL simply suppresses with the additional minus lens power. In the best of all worlds, we would have encouraged DL to undertake vision therapy. However, she is quite immature and unreliable. In checking with her previous doctor, we learn that she was totally noncompliant in attempts at vision therapy. We therefore arrive at a trial frame compromise of –0.50 sph OU for distance, which provides enough increase in clarity without making DL uncomfortable by inducing more esophoria than she can handle. In instances where more minus power is required and the patient is incapable of vision therapy to offset the binocular imbalance, base-out prism may be used to aid fusion.

Subjective

Case History, Including Signs, Symptoms, and Visual Needs

JG is a 10-year-old boy who received his first pair of glasses 6 months ago. He is an average student who is considered intelligent but avoids doing close work other than math. The first doctor his mother took him to told her that JG was uncooperative, not reading the chart as well as he could. The second doctor said JG really did not need glasses, but she would give him a prescription that would be close to a placebo, and he might be willing to try harder. JG claims that he really is trying his best, but his eyes feel funny after reading for a little while.

Lensometry

OD: +0.25
OS: +0.50

Objective

Ocular Health Assessment

All findings normal.

Clinical Measures

	At 20 ft (6 m)	At 16 in. (40 cm)
VA (sc):	OD: 20/20 (6/6)	20/20 (6/6)
	OS: 20/30 (6/9)	20/30 (6/9)
Cover Test:	Sl esop	Sl exop
N.P.C.:	3 in./6 in. (7.5 cm/15 cm) OS out; no diplopia	
Retinoscopy/	Manifest autorefraction,*	
Autorefractor:	OD: –0.75 –0.50 × 117 (9)	
	–0.50 –0.25 × 109 (9)	
	Plano –0.25 × 96 (9)	
	OS: +0.75 –0.50 × 109 (9)	
	+1.00 –0.75 × 75 (8)	
	+0.25 –0.50 × 81 (9)	

---

*The numbers in parentheses represent the confidence interval of the autorefractor, reviewed in detail in Chapter 2.

	At 20 ft (6 m)	*At 16 in. (40 cm)*
	Cycloplegic autorefraction,	
	OD: +2.00 –0.25 × 111 (9)	
	+2.25 –0.50 × 117 (9)	
	+2.00 –0.25 × 115 (9)	
	OS: +4.00 –0.25 × 116 (9)	
	+4.00 –0.50 × 110 (9)	
	+4.00 –0.50 × 119 (9)	

Subjective:	OD: Plano	VA 20/20 (6/6)
	OS: +0.50 sph	VA 20/25 (6/7.5)
Phoria:	3 esop	4 esop
Base-in vergences:	6/12/10	8/14/10
Base-out vergences:	N/E	N/E
Accom. Amplitude:	9 diopters	
Neg. Rel. Accom.:	N/E	
Pos. Rel. Accom.:	N/E	
Fused X-Cyl.:	N/E	
Stereo:	40 seconds of arc (Randot)	

Assessment

Latent hyperopic anisometropia with mild refractive amblyopia.

Plan

With the amount of latent hyperopia JG has, it is understandable that he has difficulty reading the Snellen chart with one or both eyes, particularly when he is tired. He really is trying his best but it is hard for him to sustain accommodation at near for any considerable period of time. As it turns out, the prescription that the second doctor gave JG was insightful and, when used, serves as more than a placebo.

Low plus lens power can have a significant impact on near vision performance and symptoms. Given JG's manifest versus cycloplegic refractive profile, the low power near prescription, with slightly more plus in the left eye, appears to be a good starting point. Although we strongly encouraged JG's parents to have him participate in a vision therapy program in our office, they were unable to make that commitment. When we spoke about doing a home-based vision therapy program, they decided that they would rather try the spectacle lens approach first. JG had not been wearing the glasses because his mother understood the second doctor to mean that a placebo prescription should be used as little as possible. We therefore encourage JG to wear his lens prescription for all near-point tasks, including computers, video games, schoolwork, and any form of reading, writing, or hobby. We also tell him to wear his glasses for near work right away, instead of waiting until his eyes feel funny.

JG returns to our office 3 months later and reports feeling significantly better when doing close work. His school grades have begun to improve, particularly in subjects that involved reading. Unaided visual acuities are 20/20 (6/6) through each eye at distance and near, and his manifest autorefraction is

```
OD:  +1.00 –0.25 × 107 (9)
     +1.25 –0.25 × 109 (9)
     +1.25 –0.25 × 97 (9)
OS:  +3.75 –0.25 × 131 (9)
     +4.00 –0.25 × 135 (9)
     +4.00 –0.25 × 129 (9)
```

Because JG is doing well, we keep his lens prescription and its usage the same. He returns to our office for a progress evaluation 6 months later, doing very well with all school subjects. Unaided visual acuity still is 20/20 (6/6) OD and 20/20 –2 (6/6 –2) OS. However, JG's manifest autorefractor findings show some regression toward accommodative excess, as follows:

```
OD:  –1.00 –0.25 × 53 (9)
     –0.50 –0.25 × 133 (9)
     –0.50 sphere (9)
OS:  +2.00 –0.75 × 128 (9)
     +2.25 –0.25 × 173 (9)
     +1.75 –0.25 × 113 (9)
```

JG admits that since he is doing so much better, he does not feel it is important to wear his glasses consistently. We explain to him that consistent use of the glasses at near has affected his vision the way dental retainers affect teeth: They are important for decreasing the chances that he would regress.

Six months later, JG returns for another progress evaluation and still has the same unaided visual acuity. His manifest autorefraction is as follows:

OD: Plano –0.50 × 172 (9)
  Plano –0.50 × 153 (9)
  –0.25 sphere (9)
OS: +3.00 –0.25 × 139 (8)
  +3.00 –0.50 × 149 (9)
  +2.50 –0.25 × 149 (9)

It has been 3 years since we first evaluated JG, and he has remained stable for the last three 6-month intervals. Certainly, there are similar cases where either vision therapy or a progressive addition lens might be required to address the refractive difference between left and right eyes. It is fortunate that JG's symptoms, and the stability of his condition, could be managed with low-plus single-vision lenses. The outcome reflects our clinical experience that it is better to start with simple solutions and take complex approaches as needed.

Subjective

Case History, Including Signs, Symptoms, and Visual Needs

AN is a teenager under the care of another optometrist. At his wit's end with that practitioner, he asks us for a second opinion. He is a well-rounded scholar/athlete, who excels at soccer. Before giving you more background, here is the spectacle lens prescription given him.

Lensometry

OD: –2.00 –1.25 × 180   5 BO OD
OS: –1.75 sphere   5 BO OS

Through this prescription, AN's visual acuity is 20/40 –2 (6/12 –2) OD and 20/20 –1 (6/6 –1) OS. AN's chief complaint is that he experiences double vision when he puts on the glasses. He tells us that he feels no problem with double vision without the glasses. The only thing he notices is that his vision is getting blurred at a distance, and his father is concerned that AN could not identify road signs at as far a distance as he could. AN had eye muscle surgery as a child; and each time he returned to the surgeon for examination, his parents were told that everything was fine. The optometrist who referred AN said that initially he was pleased with the glasses but then reported seeing double with them. She then tried to fit him with contact lenses, including rigid gas-permeable lenses because of his narrow palpebral apertures, but this was not successful.

Objective

Ocular Health Assessment
All findings are normal.

Clinical Measures

		At 20 ft (6 m)	At 16 in. (40 cm)
VA (unaided):	OD:	20/125 (6/38)	20/60 (6/18)
	OS:	20/80 (6/24)	20/20 (6/6)
Cover Test:		20$^\Delta$ RET	25$^\Delta$ RET'
N.P.C.:		N/E	
Retinoscopy/	OD:	−2.25 −1.00 × 180	
Autorefractor:	OS:	−1.50 sphere	
Subjective:	OD:	−1.75 −1.25 × 180	VA 20/40 −1 (6/12 −1)
	OS:	−1.75 sphere	VA 20/20 (6/6)
Phoria:		Suppr	Suppr
Base-in vergences:		Suppr	Suppr
Base-out vergences:		X/12/8	X/14/6
Accom. Amplitude:		N/E	
Neg. Rel. Accom.:		N/E	
Pos. Rel. Accom.:		N/E	
Fused X-Cyl.:		N/E	
Stereo:		No random dot stereo perceived	

Assessment

Constant right esotropia with amblyopia, and bilateral myopia.

Plan

It seems that the referring optometrist's efforts had been directed toward both fully compensating AN's myopia and trying to get him more passively aligned by incorporating prism. Because he is well adapted through central suppression of the right eye, it appears that attempts to make AN more binocular are well intentioned but counterproductive. The focus in this case should be on addressing the family's concern, which is affording AN better distance clarity for his driver's education course. Therefore, we decide to leave AN's right lens at plano and let him continue to use the right eye for peripheral awareness. Incorporating the full minus distance lens power into AN's prescription stimulates more eso, so we concentrate on a trial lens power that would noticeably improve distance clarity yet not induce double vision or discomfort. Based on trial lens responses, we change AN's lens prescription to plano OD and −0.75 sphere OS, and he subsequently wore this prescription successfully when driving.

Subjective

Case History, Including Signs, Symptoms, and Visual Needs

PA is a 44-year-old manager of a cosmetics company who reports difficulty in doing near work comfortably. She had received prescription lenses, which she was told to use for either distance or near, depending on where and when she felt she was having difficulty. She finds them of little benefit in doing desk work.

Lensometry

OD: $+0.50 -1.00 \times 97$
OS: $+0.50 -0.75 \times 78$

Objective

Ocular Health Assessment

Retinal atriovenous malformation of the right optic disk, not contributory to the case, with other eye health findings normal.

Clinical Measures

	At 20 ft (6 m)	At 16 in. (40 cm)
VA (unaided):	OD: 20/25 +1 (6/75 +1)	20/30 (6/9)
	OS: 20/20 –2 (6/6 –2)	20/30 (6/9)
Cover Test:	Ortho	Apx 10 exop
N.P.C.:	4 in./8 in. (10 cm/20 cm) OD out	
Retinoscopy/	OD: +0.75 –1.25 × 84	
Autorefractor:	OS: +0.75 –1.00 × 95	
Subjective:	OD: +0.50 –1.00 × 85	VA 20/20 (6/6)
	OS: +0.50 –1.00 × 95	VA 20/20 (6/6)
Phoria:	Ortho	10 exop
Base-in vergences:	N/E	N/E
Base-out vergences:	N/E	X/12/2
Accom. Amplitude:	N/E	
Neg. Rel. Accom.:	N/E	
Pos. Rel. Accom.:	N/E	
Fused X-Cyl.:	+1.25	
Stereo:	N/E	

Assessment

Early presbyopia with convergence insufficiency.

Plan

Prescription given for near only:

OD: +1.25 –1.00 × 85 /1$^\Delta$ BI
OS: +1.25 –1.00 × 95/ 1$^\Delta$ BI

PA is comfortable with her distance vision and feels no need for a lens prescription. However, she notices little difference at near in her ability to focus because the spherical equivalent of the prescription does not afford her any significant amount of plus lens power required for her presbyopia. In addition to the help she needs for accommodation, PA has low compensating ranges at near in regard to her exophoria, including a low recovery value. This limits her ability to sustain near work comfortably. We discuss the option of vision therapy in addition to a near-point prescription, and PA elects to try near-point lenses with a small amount of base-in prism before pursing additional treatment. At last report, she is very pleased with the prescription lenses and her ability to sustain near work comfortably.

Although earlier in this chapter we demonstrated ways of calculating initial lens prescriptions incorporating prism, with experience we tend to derive powers with high probability for improving the patient's symptoms and performance. Particularly when time and patient flow are precious commodities, patients welcome empirically derived prescriptions. In PA's case, we do not want to rock the boat by increasing the plus lens power at near excessively. By holding trial lenses over her habitual lens prescription, we arrive at a comfortable balance and range for desk work including computer needs.

Regarding the prism incorporated, we usually prescribe a total of 2 prism diopters base-in at near as the initial power for convergence insufficiency patients. We explain that we are going to include a mild prescription that will enable the eyes to work together more comfortably. Even if a higher amount of prism would be calculated based on Sheard's criterion or fixation dispar-ity findings, we initially prescribe conservatively. In our clinical experience, a horizontal prism of less than 2 prism diopters rarely is appreciated by patients as making a difference in symptoms.

Subjective

Case History, Including Signs, Symptoms, and Visual Needs
JD, a 47-year-old nursing home administrator, is a neighbor of the optometric physician who referred her. She was in a car accident several years ago but reports having had difficulty reading that is virtually lifelong. She describes herself as always having been a hands-on learner. When she was younger, she had numerous read-ing tutors who she lied to. They would ask her if she understood her lessons, and she would say yes when she really did not. JD learned to read just well enough to make it through college and graduate school in social work, but she avoided reading at all costs. Although never formally diagnosed as dyslexic, she has character-

istic inversions and transpositions of letters and numbers, which persist to this day. Recently, she has been making errors in number and letter identification and sequence that has caused significant problems in computer data entry, phone numbers, and so on. She notes that, when there are spaces between numbers or letters, such as a social security number with hyphens, she is more accurate. With a longer string of numbers or letters without spacing, the array appears to become jumbled and more errors occur. Her family and coworkers have become increasingly less sympathetic to her plight, and she initially came to determine whether she might have a visual problem that had been overlooked.

Lensometry (near prescription)
OU: +2.00

Objective

Ocular Health Assessment
All findings normal.

Clinical Measures

	At 20 ft (6 m)	At 16 in. (40 cm)
VA (unaided):	OD: 20/20 (6/6)	20/50 (6/15)
	OS: 20/20 (6/6)	20/50 (6/15)
Cover Test:	Ortho	Sl esop
N.P.C.:	2 in./4 in. (5 cm/10 cm) OS out	
Retinoscopy/	OD: +0.25 –0.25 × 93	
Autorefractor:	OS: +0.50 –0.25 × 15	
Subjective:	OD: +0.25 sphere	VA 20/20
	OS: +0.25 sphere	VA 20/20
Phoria:		
Lateral:	Ortho	8 esop
Vertical:	N/E	Ortho
Base-in vergences:	N/E	X/12/6
Base-out vergences:	N/E	X/12/8
Accom. Amplitude:	N/E	
Neg. Rel. Accom.:	N/E	
Pos. Rel. Accom.:	N/E	
Fused X-Cyl.:	+1.75	
Stereo:	N/E	

Assessment

Convergence excess and presbyopia.

Plan

We write a new prescription for JD to have her optometric physician change, which preserves the +2.00 sphere OU but incorporates 2 prism diopters base out in each lens. In contrast with the previous example of convergence insufficiency, we want to give JD a jump-start with prism that would give her more visual stability at near. In her case, it is not a matter of being able to sustain focus comfortably over time. Rather, her near phoria is significant enough and her vergence range unstable enough that some of her letter and number misidentifications could be directly attributed to her visual inefficiency.

How do we know this? We use Halberg clips to trial frame the prism over her current reading glasses. Without advising her that we are conducting a trial, we first put the prisms in the base-in direction, which is the opposite direction required for compensation. In reading a small section of telephone book print, JD's errors increase. We reverse the direction of the prism to base out, and JD reads with greater accuracy and fluency. We will further comanage JD's case with the referring optometric physician by encouraging her to undertake vision therapy, which we will monitor.

Subjective

Case History, Including Signs, Symptoms, and Visual Needs

Patient AK is a 19 year old with anisometropia and a "V" pattern exotropia. To demonstrate the longitudinal management of this case with lenses alone, we now dispense with the template of the previous cases and review only the pertinent findings observed on successive visits to our office.

We first examined AK 14 years ago, when she was 5 years old. AK was detected as having a difference in acuity between the left and right eyes during a vision screening. At that time, her unaided visual acuity was 20/25 (6/7.5) with the right eye and 20/30 (6/9) with the left eye. Subjective refraction was +0.50 sphere OD and +1.50 sphere OS, which provided 20/20 (6/6) visual acuity with either eye. We also noted a "V" pattern exotropia, in which exotropia was exhibited in upgaze, with esophoria in downgaze. In primary gaze, AK was close to orthophoria laterally, and had 3 prism diopters of vertical imbalance. However, since she had no head tilt or turn and was able to fuse effectively in primary and downgaze, we decided not to incorporate any prism into her lens prescription. We prescribed the subjective refraction, and although we encouraged vision therapy, AK's mother did not follow through.

AK returned 1 year later, and her mother reported that she was wearing the glasses for all near tasks. Her visual acuity through the prescription remained 20/20 (6/6) with each eye at distance and near. Her near-point phoria was 2^Δ exo and 3^Δ right hyper, and she was able to achieve 40 seconds of arc on random dot stereopsis testing at her Harmon distance. Retinoscopy findings had increased to +1.50 sphere OD and +2.00 sphere OS. Near vergence ranges taken with a prism bar through this power were $16^\Delta/12^\Delta$ BO and $12^\Delta/8^\Delta$ BI. Based on trial frame responses and in the interest of better binocular balance, we changed AK's prescription to

OD: +1.00 sphere
OS: +1.50 sphere

One year later, AK returned with binocular alignment and phoria values similar to the previous year, but she was not reliable on random dot stereopsis testing. On retinoscopy, we now found that the anisometropia had reversed, with +2.00 sphere OD and +1.50 OS. To pursue isometropia, we changed her prescription to

OD: +1.50 sphere
OS: +1.50 sphere

This afforded a comfortable 20/20 (6/6) visual acuity at distance and near through both eyes. AK returned each year, and her binocular profile gradually changed. Her mother reported that she was an avid reader and an excellent student, with no visual complaints.

By age 11, AK began to exhibit convergence insufficiency superimposed on the "V" pattern exotropia. In primary gaze, she was orthophoric horizontally at distance, measured 12 prism diopters of exophoria at near, which easily decompensated into an intermittent exotropia on delayed cover testing. In primary gaze, she had 4 prism diopters of right hyperphoria at distance and near. At this point, we implemented vision therapy for convergence insufficiency, which was successful in restoring a more normal convergence profile in primary gaze at near, as well as in moderate downgaze. We reduced the phoria to 6 exo in primary gaze and 2 exo in downgaze at near, with well-balanced fusional vergence ranges.

One year later, AK returned stating that she had stopped wearing the glasses and actually felt better with them off than on. Her mother presumed that AK was just becoming more self-conscious about her appearance in glasses. Unaided visual acuities remained at 20/20 (6/6) OD and OS at distance and near. Her fusion and phoria profile was stable. However, her refractive status had changed, and retinoscopic findings were +2.00 sphere OD and +0.25 –0.50 × 180 OS. Based on nearpoint retinoscopy and trial framing, we prescribed new lenses for AK, as follows:

OD: +1.25 sphere
OS: +0.50 sphere

AK returned the following year, comfortable using her lens prescription at times when she anticipated sustained close work. Retinoscopy values were +2.50 sphere OD and +0.75 –0.50 × 180 OS. We did not change the lens prescription. The next year, AK's retinoscopy values were +3.00 sphere OD and +1.00 –0.25 × 180 OS. Based on trial framing and in an attempt to tip the scales back toward isometropia, we wrote a new lens prescription of +1.00 sphere OU for near. The following year, AK returned and advised us that she had not changed her lens prescription. Retinoscopy remained relatively unchanged at +3.00 sphere OD and +0.75 sphere OS.

Some important clinical features in the timeline of this case are as follows:

1. There can be some lability in a child's refractive profile, and the clinician should attempt to encourage isometropia when possible.

2. Noncomitant strabismus does not necessarily require prismatic compensation or vision therapy when the patient is asymptomatic and high achieving.
3. It is speculative as to what extent the binocular vision profile is interrelated with the refractive profile.
4. Convergence insufficiency, or even pseudoconvergence insufficiency, may coexist with noncomitant strabismus and vertical phorias. When considering prism or vision therapy, the practitioner should first observe what effect, if any, plus lenses have on the convergence profile. Some cases, although not AK, require an add to obtain the best balance between distance and near vision needs.

Noncomitant strabismus in the form of intermittent exotropia in upgaze usually presents no functional vision problems. For children, the most common complaint relates to intermittent blur when switching fixation from the desk, which is in downgaze, to the blackboard, which is in relative upgaze. This underscores the importance of having an appropriate lens prescription in place that affords a good balance between distance and near focusing.

References

1. Koch R. *The 80/20 Principle: The Secret of Achieving More with Less.* New York: Currency-Doubleday, 1998.
2. Grisham JD. Treatment of binocular dysfunctions. In: CM Schor, KJ Ciuffreda (eds). *Vergence Eye Movements: Basic and Clinical Aspects.* Boston: Butterworth–Heinemann, 1983: 616–618.
3. Rosenfeld M. Refractive status of the eye. In: WJ Benjamin (ed). *Borish's Clinical Refraction.* Philadelphia: Saunders, 1998: 10.
4. Press LJ. Lenses and behavior. *J Optom Vis Devel.* 1990;21: 5–17.
5. Birnbaum MH. *Optometric Management of Nearpoint Vision Disorders.* Boston: Butterworth–Heinemann, 1993:161–192.

6. Polasky M. Clinical refraction. In: KL Alexander (ed). *The Lippincott Manual of Primary Eye Care.* Philadelphia: Lippincott, 1995:190.

7. Levarotsky S, Oliver M, Gottesman N, Shimshoni M. Long-term effect of hypermetropic anisometropia on the visual acuity of treated amblyopic eyes. *Br J Ophthalmol.* 1998;82:55–58.

8. Allen MC. Vertical prism adaptation in anisometropes. *Am J Optom Physiol Opt.* 1974;51:252–259.

9. Henson DB, Dharamski BG. Oculomotor adaptation to induced heterophoria and anisometropia. *Invest Ophthalmol Vis Sci.* 1982;22:234–240.

10. Dowaliby M. *Practical Aspects of Ophthalmic Optics,* 4th ed. Boston: Butterworth–Heinemann, 2001:193–207.

11. Scheiman M, Wick B. *Clinical Management of Binocular Vision: Heterophoric, Accommodative, and Eye Movement Disorders.* Philadelphia: Lippincott, 1994:245–246, 286–287.

12. Remole A. Anisophoria and aniseikonia: Part I. The relation between optical anisophoria and aniseikonia. *Am J Optom Physiol Opt.* 1989;66:659–670.

13. Remole A. Anisophoria and aniseikonia: Part II. The management of optical anisophoria. *Am J Optom Physiol Opt.* 1989;66:736–746.

14. Dwyer P, Wick B. The influence of refractive correction upon disorders of vergence and accommodation. *Optom Vis Sci.* 1995;72:224–232.

15. Schwartz I, Shapiro A (eds). *The Collected Works of Lawrence W. Macdonald, O.D.,* Vol. 1. Santa Ana, CA: Optometric Extension Program, 1992:13–23, 90–92.

16. Goss DA. *Ocular Accommodation, Convergence, and Fixation Disparity. A Manual of Clinical Analysis,* 2nd ed. Boston: Butterworth–Heinemann, 1995:47–48, 105–108.

17. Rosner J, Rosner J. *Pediatric Optometry,* 2nd ed. Boston: Butterworth–Heinemann, 1990:492–497.

18. Caloroso EE, Rouse MW. *Clinical Management of Strabismus.* Boston: Butterworth–Heinemann, 1993:76–93.

19. Heath GG. The use of graphical analysis in visual training. *Am J Optom Physiol Opt.* 1959;36:337–350.

20. Grosvenor T. *Primary Care Optometry*, 4th ed. Boston: Butterworth–Heinemann, 2002:341.

21. Richman JE, Cron MT. *Guide to Vision Therapy*. South Bend, IN: Bernell Corporation, 1987:17–18.

22. Birnbaum MH. Nearpoint visual stress: Clinical implications. *J Am Optom Assoc*. 1985;56:480–490.

23. Rundstrom MM, Eeperjesi F. Is there a need for binocular vision evaluation in low vision? *Ophthal Physiol Opt*. 1995;15:525–528.

24. London R. Passive treatments for early onset strabismus. In: MM Scheiman (ed). *Problems in Optometry*, Vol 2, No. 3. Philadelphia: Lippincott, 1990:480–495.

25. Rutstein RP, Marsh-Tootle W, London R. Changes in refractive error for exotropes treated with over-minus lenses. *Optom Vis Sci*. 1989;66:487–491.

26. Cotter SA (ed). *Clinical Uses of Prism: A Spectrum of Applications*. St. Louis: Mosby, 1995.

27. Steinman SB, Steinman BA, Garzia RP. Foundations of Binocular Vision: A Clinical Perspective. New York: McGraw-Hill, 2000:64.

28. Saladin JJ. Horizontal prism prescription. In: SA Cotter (ed). *Clinical Uses of Prism: A Spectrum of Applications*. St. Louis: Mosby, 1995:109–146.

29. Rutstein RP, Eskridge JB. Studies in vertical fixation disparity. *Am J Optom Physiol Opt*. 1986;63:639–644.

30. Griffin JR, Grisham JD. *Binocular Anomalies: Diagnosis and Vision Therapy*. Boston: Butterworth–Heinemann, 1995:479.

31. Hock DR, Coffey B. Effects of yoked prism on spatial localization and stereo-localization. *J Behav Optom*. 2000;1:143–148.

32. Remole A. Dynamic spectacle magnification versus Prentice's rule and thin lens approximations. *Practical Optometry*. 1999;10:246–251.

33. Mandell RB. *Contact Lens Practice: Hard and Flexible Lenses*, 2nd ed. Springfield, IL: Charles C Thomas, 1974:339.

34. Milder B, Rubin ML. *The Fine Art of Prescribing Glasses without Making a Spectacle of Yourself*. Gainesville, FL: Triad Publishing, 1978:290–291.

35. Veronneau-Troutman S. *Prisms in the Medical and Surgical Management of Strabismus.* St. Louis: Mosby, 1994:110.
36. Tamkins SM, Greene L, Erbe L. Accommodative and binocular vision status after excimer laser in situ keratomileusis (LASIK). *Optom Vis Sci.* 1999;76(12S):147.
37. Schlange DG. Binocular dysfunction secondary to LASIK: A case report. *Optom Vis Sci.* 2000;77(12S):101.

CHAPTER 8

Refractive Care and Contact Lenses

As indicated in the Preface and Introduction, our purpose in writing this book has been to contribute conventional wisdom and clinical pearls in refractive management that we do not often see in print. With the plethora of periodicals, journal articles, textbooks, and continuing education lectures that address contact lenses, it would be presumptuous of us to feel that a chapter devoted to the subject is necessary in a book of this nature. This chapter therefore is brief, limited to a commentary on select refractive care issues faced by clinicians engaged in a primary care rather than a specialty contact lens practice. We do not address any niche product issues or discuss lens materials in relation to corneal physiology or eye health. We also do not present case examples in the template form of other chapters, as the issues in deriving lens prescriptions are similar to what is addressed topically in the chapters on myopia, hyperopia, astigmatism, presbyopia, and binocular vision. Rather, we concentrate on the contact lens as a refractive modality, in contrast with spectacle lens correction.

Another area not covered in this chapter, or in this book for that matter, is corneal topography. We view the role of corneal topography as most relevant to the physical characteristics of contact lens fit and only secondarily to the derivation of a lens prescription. As a contemporary confluence of keratometry and fluorescein pattern analysis, corneal topography can be very useful in troubleshooting and problem solving. Corneal topography is vital in following orthokeratology or keratoconus patients, and its use prior to refractive surgery is commonplace. We take the position however that, at the primary care level, the use of corneal topography is not integral to determination of a contact lens prescription. Our perspective is based in part on having a corneal topography unit installed in the office of one of the authors, with appropriate staff training, and taking measurements on a variety of patients for a 60-day period. We decided not to keep the instrument because we did not envision that it would alter the way we analyze the patient or design lenses. However, we leave the door open to the possibility that this perspective will change in the future.

Spherical Soft Lenses

Soft (hydrogel) spherical contact lenses are the mainstay of most primary care practices. A spherical contact lens typically provides good visual acuity for patients with spherocylindrical refractive errors up to 0.75 diopter. Therefore, when initially fitting a patient with a low amount of astigmatism, we always try a spherical lens first to establish whether or not it will provide acceptable visual acuity. Spherical lenses of relatively greater thickness tend to mask more astigmatism through the resulting tear layer between the back surface of the lens and the front surface of the cornea. Our clinical experience has been that patients sometimes are happy with their visual acuity even when the residual cylinder measured in overrefraction is as high as 1.25 diopters. Certainly, if the patient is a previous contact lens wearer and happy with his or her visual acuity through a spherical lens, we think twice before encouraging a switch to a toric lens. Rigid gas-permeable (RGP) lenses have enjoyed somewhat of a resurgence, owing in part to the availability of lenses with a variety of dK or oxygen permeability values and due to interest in orthokeratology. If the refractive astigmatism and corneal astigmatism do not differ by more than 0.50 diopter, a spherical RGP lens can mask up to 2 diopters of astigmatism, providing the lens is stable on the eye.

Toric Soft Lenses

Approximately 40% of patients with spectacle lens correction have 0.75 D or more of cylinder. Although not all soft lens patients with spectacle cylinder of 0.75 D or more require toric soft lenses, about 25% of them would benefit.[1] When the measured residual astigmatism through a spherical contact lens limits the patient's best visual acuity, toric soft lenses should be used. The advent of planned replacement soft toric lenses has made this an attractive option. Several major contact lens manufacturers provide an ample variety of complementary trial lenses so that a wide array of patients can be fit with stock diagnostic lenses. For example, Bausch & Lomb (Soflens 66 Toric) and Johnson & Johnson (Acuvue Toric) provide fitting sets in a variety of spheres with cylindrical powers of 0.75, 1.25, and 1.75. The Soflens 66 Toric also has a 2.25 diopter cylinder available. The axes available are in 10° increments around the clock. This gives the practitioner an opportunity to view the lens with precise spherocylindrical power and orientation on the eye for a better-educated projection of the patient's success. When the power in either spectacle lens meridian is greater than 4 diopters, vertex distance calculations must be made to project the power requirements for the corneal plane.

The need to modify cylinder axis usually is judged by the rotation of the orientation mark on the lens. Each clock hour of rotation represents a 30° change cylinder axis location. Manufacturers of soft toric lenses supply a simple toric axis calculator. These consist of two overlapping wheels. The spectacle prescription axis wheel is dialed in first and the orientation mark wheel is set to 0 (6 o'clock position). The orientation mark wheel and spectacle axis wheel then are turned in tandem to match the orientation mark position of the lens on the eye. Rotating the orientation mark results in a new axis reading, which is the contact lens axis ordered. This follows the LARS principle, in which rotation of the orientation mark to the left (clockwise from the examiner's view) adds to or increases the axis degree and a rotation of the orientation mark to the right subtracts from or decreases the axis degree.

For example, if the spectacle lens axis is 100 and the lens is rotated 15° left, the contact lens should be ordered at axis 115°. If the lens is rotated 15° right, the axis to be ordered is 85°.

As high as the success rate is with toric soft lenses, the practitioner always should fit the lens by maximizing the spherical component and keeping the cylindrical value as low as possible to provide good acuity. The greater is the amount of cylinder in the contact lens, the greater the effects of rotational instability.[2] Among the factors that contribute to toric lens rotation or instability are these:

1. Variable lens position in different positions of gaze.
2. Lens dehydration due to poor blinking or corneal tear properties.
3. Lens dehydration due to environmental conditions.
4. Incorrect base curve.

Patients with oblique astigmatism are more difficult to fit with toric soft lenses than patients with axes within 20° of axis 90 or 180. Since the thicker meridians of oblique minus cylinders are neither parallel to nor perpendicular with movement of the upper eyelid, a translational force occurs with each blink. However, since the toric curves of many of the astigmatic soft lenses are limited to the central optic zone, the spherical skirt of the soft lens tends to provide more stability of the lens on the eye. It is one reason why toric soft lenses are fit with slightly larger diameter than their spherical counterparts.

It is important to give the lens time to settle on the eye. In many instances, if the patient feels the acuity with the lens is functional, it is best to dispense the lens and have the patient return 1 week later rather than rushing to reorder the lens with a different axis or power. When the overrefraction and the resultant power and axis of the lens do not provide the expected result, the inside curve of the lens often is at fault. A different base curve should be selected. Changing the base curve or lens type should be considered when the orientation mark on the lens is consistently rotated more than 20°.

Contact Lenses for Presbyopia

With the onset of presbyopia, we always look to prescribe the distance power that represents maximum plus lens power or minimum minus lens power. In Chapter 3 on myopia and **clinical pearl 7**, we refer to the maxim: "Keep them in the green and they'll keep you in the green." This advice on using the red/green bichrome test is given to ensure that the patient is not overplussed at distance and will be happy to pay you (green currency) for your services. However, as patients enter presbyopia, they may be willing to accept 0.25 less minus or more plus at distance in one or both eyes. When on the cusp of presbyopia, this may happily buy the patient an extra year of not having to worry about different powers for distance and near. Even when the patient is presbyopic, being able to reduce the distance prescription in one or both lenses extends the range of intermediate focus. We address these issues in more detail, and through clinical case examples, in Chapter 6 on presbyopia.

The Monovision Modality

Any contact lens correction for presbyopia, other than single-vision reading glasses used in conjunction with distance contact lenses, requires some sort of optical compromise. Having said this, the compromise involved is not much different from that required for the patient with presbyopia who must adapt to progressive addition spectacle lenses. For many years, monovision correction, in which one eye is corrected primarily for distance and the other eye primarily for near, has been a viable option for a significant number of patients.[3] The simplest and most direct way to determine how likely a patient is to adapt to a monovision contact lens correction is to determine the dominant eye for distance, and then hold a trial spectacle lens over the nondominant eye that would provide adequate near acuity. The patient who becomes queasy while sitting in the examination chair is not a particularly good candidate for monovision. If all goes well, have the patient walk around with the near add lens monocularly and then look out the window toward traffic.

Monovision is a very attractive option for patients who are just beginning to deal with presbyopia, particularly if they are well-adapted contact lens wearers.[4] There is general agreement that, as the monovision add effect increases, the probability for success diminishes.[5] As reviewed in Chapter 6, some spectacle lens wearers acquire a natural form of monovision of which they are not aware in early presbyopia until the doctor points out the phenomenon to them. Therefore, when changes between the two eyes are relatively gradual, the patient has an easier time adapting. Consider the following two scenarios. Each patient is at age 52, having entered presbyopia 10 years ago with a distance correction of minus 3.00 D sphere OU. Each patient now has a spectacle prescription of –3.00/+2.00 OU, with the previous spectacle prescription being –3.00/+1.75.

Patient A, with no prior contact lens wear, wishes to try monovision for the first time. The contact lens diagnostic prescription is

Dominant eye (OD): –3.00 D, yielding 20/20 (6/6) at distance
Nondominant eye (OS): –1.00 D, yielding 20/20 (6/6) at near

Patient B has been wearing contact lenses since her teens. She began monovision at age 42, with right eye (dominant) having a –3.00 D contact lens and left eye (nondominant) having a –2.25 D lens. Every 2 years, we decreased the near (OS) lens power by 0.25 to provide more add. Two years ago, her contact lens prescription was –3.00 OD and –1.25 OS, and she now perceives blur at near for very small print. Her contact lens diagnostic prescription is

Dominant eye (OD): –3.00 D, yielding 20/20 (6/6) at distance
Nondominant eye (OS): –1.00 D, yielding 20/20 (6/6) at near

It should be clear that, although the absolute powers are the same for both patients, patient A will have a difficult time adjusting to the induced difference, and patient B should ease into the new prescription effortlessly. Patient A has an induced anisometropia of 2 D from the habitual state, whereas patient B has to adjust to an additional anisometropia of only 0.25 D from her habitual state. Suppression tends to increase as the amount of monovision increases.[6] Paradoxically, the patient with preexisting fragile binocular vision or small central suppression may do surprisingly well with a process, such as monovision, that aids suppression.

The monovision modality can be coupled with astigmatic correction when necessary. Toric monovision obviously can apply when there is cylindrical correction necessary for one or both eyes. Many considerations must be taken into account in fitting monovision lenses, some of which are medicolegal in nature.[7] For example, the dominant eye usually takes the distance correction. However, when a trial spectacle lens add is held over the nondominant eye, the patient may report more subjective visual disturbance at distance than when it is switched in front of the dominant eye. Further, the patient who is right-eye dominant and the left eye is corrected for near may be more troubled by glare from oncoming headlights at night when driving. The point is that the clinician and the patient have to arrive at a comfort level as to how practical monovision is on a daily basis.

There are all kinds of permutations in arrangements for lens wear. They may be used more on a social basis so that patients can read a theater program or see a menu. The patient may have supplementary glasses that provide better task clarity for the near work environment or spectacle lenses kept in the glove compartment to enhance driving conditions. Successful experience with monovision contact lenses also may increase success with monovision refractive surgical outcomes.[8,9] Many of the issues encountered in monovision, which represent opportunities for lifestyle dispensing, were experienced by patient BK.

When we first evaluated BK in 1991, she was a 46-year-old computer training consultant and avid golfer. Her general health was excellent, with the exception of minor thyroid difficulties for which she took a mild dose of synthroid. BK had worn PMMA rigid lenses since she was a teenager but, in 1988, switched to soft lenses even though she was asymptomatic. When she presented for examination, BK wore the following lenses:

OD: B&L Optima II −1.25
OS: B&L Optima II −1.50

She also used a pair of single-vision spectacle lenses, +1.00 sphere OU, to provide clarity at near through the contact lenses. However, she noticed that she could read smaller print with her lenses removed than with the contact lens/reading glasses combination. She suspected that she needed stronger reading glasses. Her distance vision was generally good, but BK complained of intermittent haze. We found that, while the lenses centered and moved well, they were heavily coated with mucous. BK claimed to be compliant with lens cleaning regimens.

A friend who was successful with the monovision lens modality referred BK to our office, and she wondered if she could be corrected in this manner. Using the sighting test, BK tested as being left-eye dominant. However, when we put a lens for distance on the left eye only, she was not comfortable with the distance/ near balance. We switched the lens to the right eye, and BK was pleased with her vision. We allowed the left eye to remain uncorrected for distance, which provided her with a –1.50 add for near.

BK returned 1 week later, stating that she was generally pleased with the arrangement but insecure about driving at night or in unfamiliar areas under monovision conditions. We prescribed spectacle lenses to be used over her contact lenses for distance, as follows:

OD: Plano
OS: –1.50 sphere

One month later BK returned, reporting that she was generally pleased with the monovision fit of the lens on her right eye only. However, when looking over someone's shoulder to instruct the trainee on the computer, she needed to lean closer to the screen to focus clearly. This posed some logistical problems. We determined that, at the distance BK was fixating over someone's shoulder to the screen, an intermediate add would be ideal. Since she still had the need to focus on print with the left eye, we arrived at a "task" spectacle lens overcorrection for her computer training environment of

OD: +0.50 sphere
OS: Plano

At this juncture, BK has

1. A single contact lens distance correction OD, with OS uncorrected, providing reasonably good near acuity.
2. Supplemental glasses for smaller print (over-the-counter reading glasses).
3. Supplemental glasses for driving that compensate the OS myopia.
4. Supplemental glasses for working that provide intermediate clarity for OD.

BK returned 3 months later, and since it was summertime, she was golfing more than ever. She noticed that her ability to "read the green" was not as effective with her monovision arrangement as it had previously been when both eyes were corrected for distance. (This provides yet another twist on the advice to "keep them in the green and they'll keep you in the green.") We had BK bring her clubs to the office and set up her artificial green. She wanted to preserve a little bit of near vision for keeping score, so we found an effective compromise by giving her a trial contact lens of –0.75 for the OS. This provided a meaningful increase in her ability to localize at distance and helped her overall function on the course. Although this added a fourth combination to BK's refractive potpourri, she was very accepting and appreciative of the various options.

All remained relatively uneventful for several years. By 1994, BK's distance refraction had changed to –1.00 sphere OU, which necessitated a modification of her refractive combinations, as follows:

1. Distance contact lens reduced to –1.00 D OD.
2. Contact lens for golf reduced to –0.50 D OD.
3. Distance spectacle overcorrection for driving was reduced to –1.00 sphere OS (OD remained plano).
4. For intermediate distances, BK no longer needed a spectacle lens overcorrection. She could see reasonably well with the left eye by not wearing the contact lens (effectively providing a +1.00 add).

5. BK increased the strength of her over-the-counter reading glasses to +1.25.

In 1997, BK advised us that she has never really liked soft lenses as much as hard lenses. We refit her right eye with a Fluoroperm RGP lens, and she was pleased. At her examination in 1999, BK reported that she felt her vision had changed. Her distance refraction now was

OD: −0.75 sphere
OS: −0.50 sphere

She also noted that it had become easier to focus at distance with her left eye when her lens was out. Since her "golfing lens" for the left eye was a −0.50, we simply told BK to wear her golf lens as the new distance correction and reduced the power of her right lens to −0.75, to be used as needed. When the lens was not used on the right eye, BK had intermediate clarity, which still was satisfactory for computer instruction. She was able to read small print well enough for her needs, at age 54, with a pair of over-the-counter +1.25 magnifiers. This gave her a net effect of +2.00 at near through her right eye when the lens was not being used. She also obtained a pair of +1.75 magnifiers that she kept in the glove compartment for use when she had both distance contact lenses on for driving and had to refer to small printed directions.

The results of BK's examination in 2000 showed that her vision was subjectively stable. Her spectacle refraction for 20/20 (6/6) acuity at distance in each eye was

OD: −0.75 sphere
OS: Plano −0.50 × 75

Her visual acuity at distance with the −0.50 contact lens on the left eye still was a comfortable 20/20 and overrefraction was plano. BK asked us if we thought she was a good candidate for LASIK, because she was getting tired of wearing contact lenses. We told her emphatically no. First, the left eye still afforded her reasonable intermediate vision, and nothing would be gained by targeting a plano refraction for that eye. Second, the left eye had such a negligible refraction that she would risk having poorer uncorrected distance acuity with a surgical procedure than her current acuity without a lens or spectacle correction for that left eye.

The Multifocal Modality

A significant number of multifocal contact lens designs have proliferated, with the majority being of a rotationally symmetric design. Benjamin and Borish provide an extensive discussion about the optical principles of multifocal contact lenses, to which interested readers are referred.[10] Many primary care practitioners had shied away from bifocal contact lenses, preferring to wait until designs become available that are more predictable and present less of an optical compromise between distance and near vision needs.[11] We are firmly in that camp, opting to refer interested patients to optometric colleagues who specialize in contact lenses, including bifocal and keratoconic lenses. As with toric soft contact lenses, the soft bifocal contact lens market was aided considerably by the introduction of planned replacement bifocal lenses with ample diagnostic lenses to permit a realistic in-office trial. To date, there is no planned replacement toric soft bifocal lens, which limits the range of patients who can use this lens.

Two commonly used planned replacement multifocal lenses are the Acuvue Bifocal and the Ciba Focus Progressive. The Acuvue bifocal is available in add powers from +1.00 to +2.50 in 0.50 steps. As with other rotationally symmetric design lenses, the optics are more compromised as the add power increases. An add greater than the minimum amount necessary may enhance near vision but blur distance vision. For that reason, we typically try an add of lesser power first. If the patient has a +1.50 spectacle lens add, the +1.00 add bifocal contact lens should be selected as the initial diagnostic lens. With both diagnostic lenses in place, the practitioner and patient agree on the need for additional clarity at distance or near. If a high percentage of the patient's day is spent on near work, he or she may be more interested in maximizing near visual acuity. With diagnostic lenses in place, if near acuity is fine but distance is troublesome, the practitioner can have the patient hold a –0.25 trial lens over the dominant eye. When the practitioner intentionally underplusses the bifocal add in one eye to favor distance acuity, and the nondominant eye has the full add power for near vision, we have a modified form of monovision. When the need for distance vision is more acute than near vision, the patient can have a less modified version of monovision in which the dominant eye has a single-vision lens correction for distance, and the bifocal lens is used only for the nondominant eye.

To illustrate the possible scenarios, we use a patient with a contact lens spherical equivalent refraction of –4.00 sphere OU with OD dominant and a tentative add of +2.00 OU. We put Acuvue Bifocal lenses on with power –4.00/+2.00 OU.

Scenario 1. Blurred distance vision; near vision okay.
Option 1: Decrease add of dominant eye by 0.50
OD: –4.00/+1.50
OS: –4.00/+2.00
Result: Distance vision better, but not enough; near vision okay.
Option 2: Increase distance power of dominant eye by 0.25
OD: –4.25/+1.50
OS: –4.00/+2.00
Result: Satisfactory; there is an intermediate step where one could increase the distance power of the dominant eye by 0.25 diopter and maintain the same add, which would result in a lens power of –4.25/+2.00. Another option is to see if the same steps taken with the dominant eye provide any help when attempted with the nondominant eye.

Scenario 2. Blurred near vision; distance vision okay.
Option 1: Decrease minus in distance portion of nondominant eye
OD: –4.00/+2.00
OS: –3.75/+2.00
Result: Near vision better but not enough; distance vision okay
Option 2: Increase add in nondominant eye
OD: –4.00/+2.00
OS: –3.75/+2.50

Result: Satisfactory; if more plus is needed in front of the left eye, we can further reduce the minus lens power of the nondominant eye at distance, for a more modified monovision effect.

The optics of the Ciba Focus Progressive lens are entirely different from the Acuvue Bifocal lens. It is a front-surface aspheric center-near design rather than a concentric distance-center design. There are no multiple add powers from which to select. Rather, the initial lens is selected according to the following formula:

$$P = (SER) + \frac{add}{2}$$

where P is the initial power of the lens, SER is the spherical equivalent refraction, and the add is the target spectacle lens add. For example, if the SER is –4.00 and the patient's habitual spectacle add is +2.00, the initial lens selected is a –3.00. As alluded to earlier, if the SER is more minus than the SER of the patient's current spectacle lens or contact lens correction and the patient is satisfied with that distance lens correction, do not initially increase the minus or reduce the plus lens value of the SER.

When dealing with any type of presbyopic lens power refinement, we use loose trial lenses in 0.25 diopter lens increments, in an ascending or descending staircase method, held in front of the contact lens. The phoropter is not used, because we want the patient to make visual judgments within the space that he or she normally functions, and the refinement always is done with both eyes viewing. If he or she does a considerable amount of computer work, we will position the patient in front of a computer and conduct the loose trial lens refinement. If concern relates to driving, we have the patient look out the office window toward traffic and road signs. Returning to the example, we assume the initial Focus Progressive lens selected is –3.00 for each eye. If the patient is right-eye dominant, and reports that the computer is not as clear as is required, we hold a +0.25 trial lens over the left eye. If that improves near focusing and distance still is satisfactory, a –2.75 lens is then selected for the left eye. If additional near power is necessary, we can either reduce the right lens to –2.75 or reduce the left lens further to –2.50.

When working with bifocal contact lenses, make small incremental changes in one or both eyes. However, do not frustrate or confuse the patient by making frequent small changes during the trial lens process.[12] Often, it is better to allow the patient more adaptation time than to present a three-ring circus of trial lenses. Ultimately, the patient may have to make some visual compromises to wear bifocal contact lenses, and we must come to an agreement about what is in the patient's best interest.

Whether monovision, modified monovision, or bifocal contact lenses ultimately are successful depends on the visual desires and needs of the patient. Some patients are happy if they can function socially with a contact lens prescription and not have to use glasses. They may find it acceptable to use the lenses on a part-time basis or to have a spectacle prescription to use in conjunction with the lenses. The spectacle lens correction may be one that improves distance vision, reserved primarily for driving, or may contain a near prescription that is used for small print. Some patients will decide that their only motivation to wear contact lenses is to be free of glasses. If they must use a prescription in conjunction with their lenses, even only a small fraction of the time, they may decide that multifocal spectacle lenses are more pragmatic than contact lenses in conjunction with spectacle lenses.

Myopia Containment

The effect of rigid contact lenses on slowing the progression of myopia has long been studied since the publication of the first article that documented this observation.[13] In this section, we again consider the effect of lenses as fit on a primary care basis. A review of orthokeratology, the specialty procedure used to reverse the progression of myopia through the successive application of RGP lenses, is beyond the scope of this chapter. Interested readers may find an extensive overview of this subject elsewhere.[14]

There is consensus among clinicians that rigid contact lenses slow the progression of myopia relative to single-vision spectacle lens correction.[15,16] If so, why do clinicians not regularly employ rigid lenses as the treatment of choice for children with myopic progression? It has been speculated that one reason might be the lack of a clear mechanism as to how rigid lenses affect growth of the posterior globe.[17] The contact lens and myopia progression (CLAMP) study may help to shed more light on the predictability and mechanisms of myopia containment through RGP lenses.[18,19]

Obviously, there are pragmatic reasons why more children are not fit with rigid lenses. One is the initial difference in sensation between rigid lenses and soft lenses. Even when instilling a drop of topical anesthetic in the eye to hasten initial adaptation of the lens and facilitate the instruction of placement and removal of the lens, we find that most children have a strong preference for the feel of a soft lens. And although we can reassure the child that once he or she adapts to an RGP lens it will feel as comfortable as a soft lens, this provides little reassurance to a child whose primary motivation for contact lenses is cosmesis. Another factor to consider is sports performance. For the athletic child, soft contact lenses are less likely to dislodge or eject.

Parents express concern about the responsibility of the child in caring for the lenses and the cost of lens replacement in case of loss or damage. On both counts, soft lenses with frequent planned replacement becomes a comparatively more attractive option from a parental point of view. If children and their parents tend to favor soft lenses, can we say that soft lenses favorably influence the rate of myopic progression? From a theoretical standpoint, either soft or rigid lenses provide the same relative image magnification as compared with spectacle lenses of equivalent power, which may be one mechanism that is slowing the natural course of myopic progression.[20] However, soft lenses do not appear to be as effective as rigid lenses in controlling the rate of myopic progression. It has been suggested that some patients are susceptible to myopic creep that may be associated with dehydration of soft lenses and subsequent changes in corneal topography contributing to increased myopia.[21]

Anisometropia

In Chapter 7, we note that contact lenses may provide an advantage over spectacle lenses depending on AC/A relationships and the type of ametropia. For example, patients with hyperopia have an induced base-out prismatic demand when reading through glasses that is eliminated when switching to contact lenses.[22] Patients with accommodative esotropia also may benefit from bifocal contact lenses.

We close the chapter by reiterating our clinical experience with contact lenses versus spectacle lens correction in cases of anisometropia, alluded to in Chapter 7. Knapp's law predicts that cases of axial anisometropia have less aniseikonia when corrected at the spectacle plane rather than the corneal plane. This theoretically guides the practitioner toward fitting patients with high unilateral myopia with contact lenses rather than spectacles. However, the vertical prism imbalance induced by spectacle lenses appears to be a much greater impediment to fusion than the amount of induced aniseikonia.[23]

In this regard, we relate a simple yet elegant experiment conducted by Linksz and Stollerman.[24] Working with patients having unilateral aphakia, they speculated that the variable prismatic imbalance induced by spectacle lenses was a greater impediment to fusion than image size differences between the two eyes. To prove their point, they took the spectacle lenses and taped the surface, leaving only a 10-mm window through which the patient could view. This resulted in the patient utilizing head movements to scan the visual field rather than eye movements. When restricted to viewing in this manner, patients did not report diplopia. As soon as the viewing area was widened, the patients began to experience diplopia. They concluded that induced prismatic imbalance was indeed a greater impediment to fusion than aniseikonia.

We therefore adopted a clinical policy that every patient who would benefit from a contact lens prescription should be given the option of a contact lens trial. In no case would we avoid trying contact lenses because of a theoretical presumption that the patient would benefit more from spectacle lens correction.

References

1. White P. Contact lenses and astigmatism. *Contact Lens Spectrum.* 1997;12(8):44–49.

2. Benjamin WJ. Contact lenses: Clinical function and practical optics. In: WJ Benjamin (ed). *Borish's Clinical Refraction*. Philadelphia: Saunders, 1998:1000.

3. Josephson JE, Erickson P, Back A, et al. Monovision. *J Am Optom Assoc.* 1990;61:820–826.

4. Gauthier CA, Holden BA, Grant T, et al. Interest of presbyopes in contact lens correction and their success with monovision. *Optom Vis Sci.* 1992;69:858–862.

5. Erickson P, Farkas P. Monovision contact lens fitting: A safe and effective clinical option for presbyopes. *J Behav Optom.* 1992;5:122–126.

6. Heath DA, Hines C, Schwartz F. Suppression behavior analyzed as a function of monovision addition power. *Optom Vis Sci.* 1986;63:198–201.

7. Harris MG, Classe JG. Clinicolegal considerations of monovision. *J Am Optom Assoc.* 1988;59:491–494.

8. Jain S, Arora I, Azar DT. Success of monovision in presbyopes: A review of the literature and potential applications to refractive surgery. *Surv Ophthalmol.* 1996;40:491–499.

9. Hom MM. Monovision and LASIK. *J Am Optom Assoc.* 1999; 70:117–122.

10. Benjamin WE, Borish IM. Presbyopic correction with contact lenses. In: WJ Benjamin (ed). *Borish's Clinical Refraction*. Philadelphia: Saunders, 1998:1023.

11. Bennett ES, Henry VA. Bifocal contact lenses. In: ES Bennett, VA Henry (eds). *Clinical Manual of Contact Lenses*. Philadelphia: Lippincott, 1994:362–398.

12. Spinell MR, Silbert JA. Contact lenses: The challenge and the ecstasy. *Rev Optom.* 2000;137(12):40–48.

13. Morrison RJ. Contact lenses and the progression of myopia. *Optom Weekly.* 1956;47:1487–1488.

14. Grosvenor T, Goss DA. *Clinical Management of Myopia*. Boston: Butterworth–Heinemann, 1999:155–180.

15. Rengstorff RH. Refractive changes after wearing contact lenses. In: AJ Phillips, J Stone (eds). *Contact Lenses*, 3rd ed. Boston: Butterworth–Heinemann 1989:741.

16. Grosvenor T, Perrigin D. Perrigin J, et al. Do rigid gas permeable lenses control the progress of myopia? *Contact Lens Spectrum.* 1991;5(7):29–36.

17. Mutti DO. Can we conquer myopia? *Rev Optom.* 2001;138: 80–92.

18. Walline JJ, Mutti DO, Zadnik K. The contact lens and myopia progression (CLAMP) study early results. Paper presented at *Myopia 2000: Proceedings of the VIII International Conference on Myopia,* July 7–9, 2000, Boston.

19. Walline JJ, Mutti DO, Jones LA. The contact lens and myopia progression (CLAMP) study: Design and baseline data. *Optom Vis Sci.* 2001;78:223–233.

20. Press LJ. Control of progressive myopia. In: LJ Press, B Moore (eds). *Clinical Pediatric Optometry.* Boston: Butterworth–Heinemann, 1993:327–334.

21. Caroline P, Campbell R. Long term effects of hydrophilic contact lenses on myopia. *Contact Lens Spectrum.* 1991;5(6):68.

22. Moore BD. Pediatric contact lenses. In: BD Moore (ed). *Eye Care for Infants and Young Children.* Boston: Butterworth–Heinemann, 1997:302.

23. Moore BD. Pediatric contact lenses. In: LJ Press, B Moore (eds). *Clinical Pediatric Optometry.* Boston: Butterworth–Heinemann, 1993:242–243.

24. Linksz A, Bannon RE. Aniseikonia and refractive problems. *Int Ophthalmol Clin Refraction.* 1965;5:515–525.

CHAPTER 9

Refractive Perspectives for the Post-Refractive-Surgery Patient

If we define *refractive surgery* as the utilization of techniques that physically alter the eye or its contents, we have two general types to consider: orthokeratology and those under the specific heading of "refractive surgery." We discuss orthokeratology first, which features the selection and utilization of a rigid contact lens, more recently rigid gas-permeable lenses, with radii differing from the patient's cornea surface to achieve temporary corneal reshaping. As an example, the clinician would fit a myopic eye with a flatter base curve lens than the patient's corneal surface to physically flatten the central cornea and shorten the axial length of the eye. The "treatment" and later the "retainer" lens usually is worn during the night and removed when the patient is awake.[1] More than likely, the clinician's initial awareness that the unfamiliar patient is receiving this care should be evident during the case history. If the patient currently is under care, it usually is prudent to redirect the patient to the primary clinician. If that is not possible, with the patient's authorization, become familiar with the patient's ocular records prior to care. The more conventional refractive treatment of the orthokeratology patient requires little more information than is presented elsewhere in this book, other than the awareness that the longer the patient is without the contact lens the more likely the cornea will begin to resume its original shape. This variable makes some orthokeratology patients poor candidates for a stable refractive correction.[2,3] Obviously, the clinician must carefully investigate and be particularly observant of

239

the condition of the cornea, since treatment decisions hinge on this information.

Refractive surgery is changing constantly. In a brief period of time, we have observed the introduction of and modifications in radial keratotomy (RK), keratomileusis, keratophakia, and corneal molding with the eximer laser (PRK). Combinations and variations of these techniques also evolved. New instrumentation and improvements in surgical techniques will be introduced, older procedures will be replaced, and the comanagement role of the clinicians also will continue to evolve. However, it appears safe to speculate that, at least for the next few years, LASIK will be the standby for the majority of refractive procedures performed. LASIK has superseded other techniques because of its greater safety and predictibility.[4] In fact, LASIK has also been shown to be effective in enhancing the less-than-optimum results of other refractive surgical techniques.[5-7]

In addition, longitudinal studies will report on the long-term effects of these procedures, which will help the clinician to provide optimum care. Refractive surgery is a topic of such dimension as to have generated textbooks solely committed to all aspects of this therapy. Consistent with the scope of this book, we present a brief, somewhat introductory, survey of this topic rather than a detailed discussion. In this arena, as with the remainder of those issues within the scope of professional practice, it is essential that the practitioner keep current with the literature to best serve patients and retain the position of knowledgeable contemporary provider.

In addition to other care, many post-refractive-surgery patients require the more traditional refractive care, although typically with reduced refractive errors than in their presurgery status.[8] They differ from other patients in their case history revealing refractive surgery. The timeliness of more conventional refractive intervention (i.e., spectacle or contact lens correction) depends on the technique employed, the healing process, and the visual needs of the specific patient. Due to variability in healing rates and the influence of dry eye symptoms, it is desirable to delay prescribing spectacle lenses for a few months, if possible. This delay also allows more adaptation time for the patient to a new seeing environment. During this interval, the vast majority of patients are very pleased with the freedom from glasses or contact lenses.[9] The clinical aspects of this delay period continue to evolve with the research data and experience. As these parameters become better defined, postsurgical refractive care will parallel the issues presented elsewhere in this book.

The refractionist needs awareness of the "pearls." Patient satisfaction is determined as in the past, except that the surgical intervention sometimes confuses the issue both physiologically and psychologically. Those patients requiring a spectacle correction postsurgically initially may resist this intervention if a better nonspectacle outcome was anticipated and seek satisfaction from the surgeon. The less-than-satisfied patient may blame the referring primary care practitioner along with the surgeon, particularly if the procedure was aggressively overmarketed. All the participating clinicians may find themselves legally at risk if the patient perceives the surgery is "unsuccessful." The patient is faced with two possible approaches if additional refractive intervention is needed. The patient who prefers to consider additional surgery is best directed to revisit the surgeon for a modification procedure. This is not an unusual occurrence. If the acuity situation can be resolved with spectacle correction and the patient is amenable to this, this is the other approach. The two perspectives should be discussed with the patient. Typically, these surgical modification procedures (enhancements) are performed without an additional fee, but the advantages and disadvantages of the two choices relate to the needs and preferences of the patient and the causes of the less than desired vision. The Waring et al. study quantifying the long-term (10-year) results of radial keratotomy reports that 10% of the patients needed additional procedures, 85% had an acuity of 20/40 (6/12) or better, 60% were within 1.00 diopter of emmetropia, and 43% had a hyperopic shift with the passage of time.[10] A more recent study from the Emory Vision Correction Center of 1,028 eyes having LASIK reports that 58% had results within 0.50 diopters of the intended refraction, 90% had an uncorrected acuity of 20/40 (6/12) or better, 37% underwent enhancement, and 6% had complications.[4] A problem with longitudinal studies of new surgical procedures is that techniques and instrumentation change in the decade that longitudinal studies might require. Therefore, be aware that the standard of success identified with surgical intervention has been a distance acuity of 20/40 (6/12) or better. Few refractionists would consider this a desirable endpoint definition of clarity, and most patients with this level of acuity require spectacle correction. Many surgeons prepare the patients for less satisfactory results during the case presentation by indicating that subsequent "re-treatment" or "enhancement" procedures may be necessary 4–6 months after the original procedure. Gayton reported a 33% en-hancement rate with RK, largely with the need for additional in-cisions, deeper incisions, or reducing the central clear zone.[11]

Some causes for retreatment of the various procedures are under- or overcorrection, corneal haze with or without myopic regression, increasing myopia developing during healing, optical zones that are too small having greatest impact on night vision, and decentration of the optical area.[12]

The postsurgical patient still requires clear, comfortable, effi-cient vision just like the nonsurgical patient. A problem may arise in some situations when the surgical intervention has compromised the potential for total patient visual satisfaction. If the patient is bothered by reduced contrast sensitivity or glare, coated or ab-sorptive lenses may subjectively help. As with the more traditional patient, the clinician must listen to the patient to learn about his or her needs and expectations. The primary clinician also should con-sider discouraging those patients who may be more likely candi-dates for dissatisfaction. Some of these are visually supersensitive patients, the type who would react to small degree changes on 0.25 diopter cylinders or whose glasses never are sufficiently clean or in proper adjustment. We have all seen patients of this type.

In examining potential refractive surgical patients, the clini-cian must keep current with the literature regardless of the degree of cooperating activity with the surgeon. Experience and infor-mation are helpful in learning which refractive techniques and corrections are the most useful for specific patients. Spectacle pre-scription lens design, materials, and properties as well as the like-lihood of a contact lens recommendation may be influenced by idiosyncratic aspects of specific surgical techniques and the re-sultant outcome of the patient. This information should be well within the acquired knowledge base of the clinician.

The position of the clinician in counseling the patient whether or not to submit to refractive surgery or to later return for additional corrective surgery has to be determined on a case-by-case basis. The successful contact lens wearer who has no specific "uncorrected" acuity requirements may be best treated with the continued use of contact lenses. (We define *successful contact lens wear* by patient satisfaction, good vision, and an eye not pathologically affected by the lenses.) Unlike the more permanent results of surgery, contact lens prescriptions can be modified easily as the patient's needs change and different lens prescriptions can be designed for specific visual needs. If monovision is desired the use of contact lenses may be more desirable than surgically created monovision. Some patients with monovision are less comfortable driving at night when binocularity is compromised. With contact lenses one or both of the lenses can be removed, another lens(s) inserted, or replaced with a binocular spectacle correction for this purpose or any other reason. In a surgical situation, the surgeon must program how the patient is to function and create the appropriate outcome, which is more or less permanent, although corrective lenses can also be prescribed as an overcorrection for specific needs.

Nonetheless, the contact lens population is generally targeted as potential patients for surgical intervention, since some of the same motivations that caused them to choose contact lenses still apply. The principal motivational issues driving patients to refractive surgery typically are patients who

1. Are unhappy depending on glasses or contact lenses.
2. Have become intolerant of contact lenses.
3. Are dissatisfied with their appearance in glasses.
4. Have specific sports and lifestyle needs.
5. Have occupational requirements that require a minimum level of uncorrected visual acuity.[13]

The Initial Examination of the Potential Refractive-Surgery Patient

The examination process is much the same as with any other patient except for a different emphasis and projection. The case history might reveal the patient's interest in refractive surgery, which will set the tone for added discussion during the case summary and presentation portion of the encounter. Also some patients who might not specifically indicate that they wish refractive surgery have examination results identifying their visual needs as such that the clinician might discuss this option during the presentation of the treatment options. At that time, the practitioner is better able to discuss all the ocular issues as well as answer questions. The dialogue would reveal any ocular or systemic history that might be significant in appropriately counseling the patient. Tests relating to the general and ocular health and integrity of the eye obviously are essential for the same reason.

The refractive portion of the encounter will reveal the current refractive error as well as the corrected acuity. Obviously, the patient with an amblyopia, such as one with a best corrected vision of 20/80 (6/24) that is not improved with the pinhole, should not reasonably anticipate 20/40 (6/12) after surgery. The accommodative and binocular status of the patient is important, too. A patient with a reduced amplitude of accommodation may need a near correction after surgery, depending on the refractive outcome. The patient with a binocular problem requiring prism will lack the benefit of prism postsurgically without glasses.

As mentioned before, during the case summary and presentation portion of the visit, the results of the examination and their potential impact on refractive surgery should be explored, along with a discussion of any other options available to the patient. Along with other pearls, **clinical pearl 1**, listen to your patient, is particularly appropriate to learn the needs and wants of the patient. A poorly motivated patient might be a poor candidate for anything other than a continuation of a spectacle correction. The patient also might reveal an unreasonable expectation for refractive surgery. This is increasingly more likely in markets where there is aggressive advertising for refractive surgery.

Clinical pearl 18, which speaks to the need for the patient to adapt to the new glasses, must be altered to remind patients that they may have to adapt to an entirely new visual world.

Just as the spectacle-lens-wearing myopic patient of more than 4 diopters may report near-point symptoms when switching to contact lenses, he or she also may report this when changing from spectacle wear to refractive surgery. This is due to changes in the accommodative-vergence demand now that the optics are moved from the spectacle plane to the corneal one. Since the majority of the refractive surgery candidates have high myopic errors, those who were not wearing contact lenses may fall into this category, and this potential should be presented to them, especially if they wore glasses for near-point tasks. Adjusting to the postsurgical environment may require one or a combination of adaptations, lenses for near, prisms, or vision therapy.

Contraindications to Refractive Surgery

Refractive surgery is contraindicated in some situations. These include patients with such systemic immunologic conditions as lupus erythematosus, rheumatoid arthritis, or other collagen vascular diseases. Conditions that may compromise wound healing—diabetes mellitus and immune system deficiencies—also are reasons to pause before recommending refractive surgery. In addition, progressive myopia, as well as those ocular conditions with severe dry eyes and existing corneal disease or degenerations such as keratoconus, also might contraindicate refractive surgery. Additional situations also might give pause to the suggestion of surgery. One example of this is the possible risk associated with the postoperative use of corticosteroids with a patient having, or at risk for, glaucoma. The patient with cataracts might be dissuaded since surgical correction of the cataract with intraocular lenses in the near future might be used to compensate for refractive needs.[14]

Complications Associated with Refractive Surgery

Perhaps the most frequent complication occurs when the outcome does not produce the desired nearly emmetropic refractive condition. When the outcome is refractive, a modifying surgical procedure can be considered. A particularly unhappy category of patient is a lifelong myopic patient who is overcorrected and becomes hyperopic.

Most of the nonrefractive complications of LASIK are related to the corneal flap created by the microkeratome. A more frequent occurrence is subjective glare. According to Nordan,[15] while subjective glare has not been ignored by the surgeons, their primary focus on Snellen acuity as a measure of success has reduced this glare to a lesser priority. Irregular epithelium, corneal scars, and anterior stromal haze can lead to glare and reduce the contrast sensitivity of the patient. The prescribing of lenses that absorb or reduce glare may be beneficial.

Surgically altered corneal changes may also compromise the patient's vision. The most frequent occurrences are

1. Induced corneal astigmatism (usually irregular) either as a direct result of the surgery or when the corneal strength has been compromised.
2. Decentered optical zone diameters causing some unfocused light to fall on the retina.[15]

No procedure, not contact lenses nor surgery, is entirely risk free; and consider that refractive surgery typically is applied to a healthy eye. The patient needs to be advised of the relative risks versus the likely benefits. The potential of the patient permanently throwing away all glasses, as frequently implied in advertisements, should be presented as doubtful, particularly if their eyes change with time, as with pending presbyopia and other refractive changes. The hyperopic changes that often exist as patients become presbyopic increases this possibility. Myopic patients can be assured that their postsurgical uncorrected distance vision quite likely will be improved. Also keep in mind that most patient satisfaction studies reveal a high level of satisfaction. One report stated that more than 80% of the post-refractive-surgery patients indicated being "satisfied" or "very satisfied" with their visual acuity and refractive results.[8]

Some surgical refractive techniques compromise the potential success of postsurgical contact lenses; this too must be part of the dialogue. Therefore, some patients undergoing certain surgical procedures will not have the option of simply going back to contact lenses for additional refractive correction. This is particularly true if radial keratotomy produces a corneal topography that differs from the typical ametropia. While initially soft lenses may prove more comfortable for these patients, the development of cysts and superficial neovascularization with these lenses may result in rigid gas-permeable lenses being the material of choice after RK.[1] Although RK currently is employed less frequently, we still face patients who had this technique.

Another important issue for the primary care practitioner is the skill of the surgeon with the chosen procedure. As with all referrals, appropriate care for patients is the highest priority. While most of the issues stated in this chapter are of more direct concern to the surgeon, if the initial practitioner is to serve as a patient advocate, these items need to be addressed. The discussion also enables patients to appropriately participate in their care at all levels.

As mentioned before, the chapter is only a brief overview of the topic. We must seek all legitimate avenues of information concerning these topics.[4] The surgeons seeking referrals or their representatives may not be as objective as desired. A considerable amount of scientifically sound literature concerning refractive surgery is available.

References

1. Pasternak J. Orthokeratology. In: DT Azar (ed). *Refractive Surgery.* Stamford, CT: Appelton and Lange, 1997:617–623.
2. Polse KA, Brand RJ, Vasine DW, Schalbe JS. Corneal change accompanying orthokeratology. *Arch Ophth.* December 1983; 101:1873–1878.
3. Brand RJ, Polse KA, Schwalbe JS. The Berkeley orthokeratology study. Parts I and II. *Amer J Optom and Physiol Optics.* 1993;60(3):175–198.
4. Machat JJ, Slade SG, Probst LE. *The Art of LASIK,* 2nd ed. Thorofare, NJ: Slack Inc., 1999:3–5, 281–292.
5. Clausse MA, Boutross G, Khanjian G, Wagner C, Garabet AL. A retrospective study of laser in situ keratomileusis after radial keratectomy. *J Refrac Surg.* March–April 2001;17(suppl.): S200–S220.

6. Lipshitz I, Man O, Shemesh G, Lazar M, Loewensite A. Laser in situ keratomileusis to correct hyperopic shift after radial keratotomy. *J Cat Refrac Surgery.* February 2001;27(2): 273–276.

7. Attia WH, Alio JL, Artola A, Munez G, Shalaby A. Laser in situ keratomileusis for undercorrection and overcorrection after radial keratotomy. *J Cat Refrac Surgery.* February 2001;27 (2):267–272.

8. Ben-Sira A, Loewenstein A, Lipshitz I, Levanon D, Lazar M. Patient satisfaction after 5.0 mm photorefractive keratectomy for myopia. *J Refrac Surg.* March–April 1997;13:129–134.

9. Toczolowski J, Oles P, Zagorski A, et al. The sense of self-concept. Changes in patients after radial keratotomy. *J Refrac Surg.* March–April 2001;17:134–137.

10. Waring GO III, Lynn MJ, Azhar N, et al. Results of the prospective evaluation of the radial keratotomy (PERK) study at 10 years after surgery. *Ophthalmol.* 1991;98:1164–1176.

11. Gayton JL, Van Der Kerr M, Sanders V. Radial keratotomy enhancements for residual myopia. *J Refrac Surg.* March–April 1997;13:374–381.

12. Gartry DS, Stasiuk R, Robinson D. Prevention and management of complications of photorefractive keratectomy. In: ON Serdarevic (ed). *Refractive Surgery: Current Techniques and Management.* New York: Igaku-Shoin Medical Publishers, 1997:85–94.

13. Brint SF, Fisher CS, Johnson DG, Ashton B, Tseng P, Jackson WB. Refractive centers: Operations and management. In: ON Serdarevic (ed). *Refractive Surgery: Current Techniques and Management.* New York: Igaku-Shoin Medical Publishers, 1997:293–307.

14. Azar DT. *Refractive Surgery.* Stamford CT: Appleton and Lange, 1997:101–102.

15. Nordan LT, Complications of corneal refractive surgery: Emphasis on corneal structure. In: ON Serdarevic (ed). *Refractive Surgery: Current Techniques and Management.* New York: Igaku-Shoin Medical Publishers, 1997:281–292.

16. Hom MM. *LASIK: Clinical Comanagement.* Boston: Butterworth–Heinemann, 2001:92, 94, 100, 107.

CHAPTER 10

Refractive Care of the Patient with Diabetes

It has been stated that possibly 50% of the estimated 6.5–14 million patients in the United States having diabetes mellitus are undiagnosed. The number of undiagnosed patients results in the enormous range in the projected number of cases. Although it can occur at any age, its prevalence has been estimated to exist in 10% of the population over 60 years of age and increases to 16–20% over 80. Diabetes mellitus results in 12% of all new cases of blindness each year. Severe visual disability most frequently is the result of diabetic retinopathy, macular edema, or vitreous hemorrhage.[1] Diabetic retinopathy is the most common of the long-term serious complications of diabetes; however, having diabetes more than doubles the patient's risk of glaucoma and cataracts, as well as increases the possibility of other ocular effects, including optic nerve atrophy, increased intraocular pressure, diplopia, and rubiosis iridis. The recommended frequency of ocular examinations as well as other management guidelines for patients having diabetes are spelled out in the *AOA Clinical Practice Guideline: Care of the Patient with Diabetes Mellitus.* Among the recommendations is the need for annual dilated fundus examinations. We strongly recommended this monograph for its practical clinical guidance as well as its reference lists.[2]

We define *diabetes mellitus* as a disease characterized by hyperglycemia. While the ocular effects of the disease may fall on any aspects of the ocular system, to be consistent with the mission of this text we emphasize those related to the spectacle correction, primarily the refractive changes due to alterations in the blood sugar and, less frequently, the binocular problems relating to nerve palsy.[1,3]

Diabetes is clinically divided into two major categories: insulin-dependent diabetes mellitus (IDDM) and non-insulin-dependent diabetes mellitus (NIDDM), with the obvious difference being that insulin may not be the primary treatment in NIDDM.

The typical refractive patient with undiagnosed diabetes mellitus presents with a sudden change in vision. The most common ocular effect of diabetes is a refractive shift usually to more myopia (or less hyperopia) with elevated blood sugar levels.[3(p. 104)] Since this can take place over a short period of time, several hours to several days in acute situations, it is of particular importance to question the patient relating to the duration of awareness of a visual change. This somewhat rapid rate of change helps differentiate the refractive alteration resulting from diabetes from other refractive changes, such as the increase in myopia found with a nuclear cataract progression. Both situations produce a myopic shift.

The refractive power of the crystalline lens is a combination of its radius of curvature and index of refraction. Osmotic lens swelling due to imbibition of water reduces its refractive index while concurrently increasing its radius of curvature. In most patients, the fluid retention increasing the radius of curvature (and increasing the plus power of the lens) outweighs the reduction of the index of refraction, so more myopia predominates, but in some the reverse is true and we may find a shift toward hyperopia in some patients with uncontrolled diabetes. An example of this is patient DA.

Subjective

Case History, Including Signs, Symptoms, and Visual Needs

DA, a 42-year-old patient, reports that she "suddenly" is not seeing well at distance with her distance glasses or at near when she removes them. She had been reading without glasses but now is unable to do so unless she moves too close to the reading matter. Her present glasses (for distance only) are 2 years old and, until recently, were quite satisfactory for distance. She has been having some unusual physical symptoms recently, including increased thirst, frequent urination, and recent weight gain. She disclosed a family history of both parents having diabetes. Otherwise, she reports no aches, pain, or diplopia. The remainder of her history is unremarkable.

DA drives and watches television with glasses. She reads at 16 in. and her computer screen at work is at 24 in. (60 cm). In the past, she did not need glasses for these near tasks; removing her glasses was satisfactory. She performs data entry for an insurance company, using a computer for the entire work day.

Lensometry

For distance only,

OD: –1.75 DS
OS: –1.25 DS

Objective

Ocular Health Assessment

No signs of ocular or systemic health problems. Dilated fundus examination is performed. In keeping with the emphasis on refractive issues, we do not detail yet are aware of the need for the careful external and internal ocular examination appropriate to the diabetic patient, which includes a dilated fundus examination.

Clinical Measures

	At 20 ft (6 m)	At 16 in. (40 cm)
VA (with	OD: 20/200 (6/60)	20/20 (6/6)
prescription):	OS: 20/200 (6/60)	20/20 (6/6)
Cover Test:	Ortho	Ortho
N.P.C.:	4 in. (10 cm)/6 in. (15 cm)/ diplopia reported	
Retinoscopy/	OD: –3.75 DS	
Autorefractor:	OS: –3.25 DS	
Subjective:	OD: –3.25 –0.25 × 90	VA 20/20 (6/6)
	OS: –3.25 DS	VA 20/20 (6/6)

	At 20 ft (6 m)	*At 16 in. (40 cm)*
Phoria:	Ortho	4 exo (near)
Base-in vergences:	N/E	15/15/9
Base-out vergences:	N/E	12/12/7
Accom. Amplitude:	0.75 each eye	
Neg. Rel. Accom.:	N/E	
Pos. Rel. Accom.:	N/E	
Fused X-Cyl.:	+2.00 add, giving 20/20 (6/6) in each eye at 16 in (40 cm). Phoria through +2.00 tentative add = 6 exop	
Stereo:	N/E	

Assessment

Apparently sudden increase in myopia, suggestive of diabetes. No other signs of pathology.

Plan

1. Refer and consult with internist as soon as possible.
2. Discuss suspicions with DA.
3. If at all possible, delay implementation of a new spectacle correction. DA is advised to use her present glasses for reading and computer work and not to drive until the underlying condition is diagnosed and treatment stabilizes the condition. DA should understand that, if it is diabetes, the apparent increase in myopia will diminish shortly. In any event, the patient should return for a refractive reevaluation in 1 month and call before that if she has any questions.
4. If diabetes is confirmed the patient needs to be aware of the need (a) to follow the instructions of her physician, (b) to return yearly for a dilated fundus examination and refraction, and (c) to contact you if she has any ocular symptoms or questions.

If DA cannot function visually and there is great liklihood of refractive variations, it might be necessary to prescribe spectacles as a temporary measure. Given this situation, consider single-vision lenses as opposed to multifocals or a limited supply of disposable contact lenses. These must be dispensed with the patient understanding the probably temporary nature of the correction because of the fragility of the ocular system. The fabricating of new bifocals would be quite costly, particularly since their effectiveness likely will be short lived. In any event, DA should return for another refractive visit after her internist reports that the blood sugar has stabilized.

The care with patients having diabetes mellitus always requires counseling and consultation with the patient's internist. The sudden onset of diplopia might suggest a neurological consultation. The diplopia may be related to diabetes or some other neurological problem, so the referral must be immediate since it may be life threatening. Nerve palsy occurs in 4% of patients with diabetes, primarily affecting the III, IV, or VI cranial nerves.[3] The deviation observed depends on the nerve affected and may present with a symptom of diplopia, a compensating head tilt, and if involving the III cranial nerve, an accompanying ptosis. The initial refractive management consists of occlusion of the deviating eye or prescribing spectacle lenses with prism. Some practitioners prefer to use Fresnel Press-On Prisms, since the palsy usually is self-limiting and resolves in several months, if the blood sugar levels stabilize. The amount of prism and its direction depend on the amount and direction of the deviation. In determining the amount and direction of the prism, the minimum power and base orientation should be sufficient to allow the patient to fuse. Since the deviation usually is temporary and self-resolving, there should be a reluctance to grind the prism into a spectacle correction. However, if lenses are going to be ground, the amount of prism typically is divided between the two eyes, for cosmetic appearance and to minimize aberrations. Press-on prisms present no lens thickness problem of consequence but they diminish the acuity by several lines on the Snellen chart. The stronger the prism is, the greater this diminution. As a result, practitioner judgment should be exercised whether to divide it between the two eyes to maximize equality of the diminished vision or to place the prism on the nondominant eye. However, this process may discourage binocularity due to the differences in the corrected acuities. Another option is the temporary use of prefabricated training goggles or clip-ons that can be worn over glasses.

An example of an apparent diabetic-induced palsy follows.

Subjective

Case History, Including Signs, Symptoms, and Visual Needs

Patient DB, a 56-year-old woman, was told this morning by her physician that she has diabetes and must take insulin. Her symptoms include recent diplopia and reduced vision with her glasses at far. She reports seeing better at distance without her distance glasses, and her "bifocals are too strong for near." She presents with a head tilt. Her visual needs include driving and watching television. She wears glasses most of the time. Recently, she noticed that her distance seeing with glasses was very poor but now she can read using the distance portion of her bifocals. DB prefers to read at 16 in. (40 cm).

Lensometry
OD: +3.75 –0.75 × 90
OS: +2.75 –0.25 × 90
OU: +2.00 add

Objective

Ocular Health Assessment

Iris, pupillary reflexes, lenses, and fundus healthy (with dilation).

Clinical Measures

	At 20 ft (6 m)	At 16 in. (40 cm)
VA (no prescription):	OD: 20/200 (6/60)	N/E
	OS: 20/200 (6/60)	N/E
Cover Test:	6$^\Delta$ Rt. hypo/	6$^\Delta$ Rt. hypo/
	10$^\Delta$ XT	10$^\Delta$ XT′
N.P.C.:	N/E (no fusion)	
Retinoscopy/	OD: +1.75 –0.50 × 90	
Autorefractor:	OS: +0.75 DS	

	At 20 ft (6 m)	*At 16 in. (40 cm)*
Subjective:	OD: +1.75 –0.50 × 90	VA 20/20 (6/6)
	OS: +0.75 DS	VA 20/20 (6/6)
Phoria:	N/E	
Base-in vergences:	N/E	N/E
Base-out vergences:	N/E	N/E
Accom. Amplitude:	1.25 each eye	
Neg. Rel. Accom.:	N/E	
Pos. Rel. Accom.:	N/E	
Fused X-Cyl.:	N/E	
Plus Build-up:	+2.00 add 20/20 (6/6) each eye	
Stereo:	N/E	

Assessment

Refractive shift toward less hyperopia OU, most likely due to increased blood sugar. Nerve palsy causing diplopia also may be due to diabetes. Eyes otherwise healthy.

Plan

1. Consult patient's internist.
2. Counsel DB concerning compliance with internist's advice and educate her concerning the need for annual eye examinations (with dilation) as well as remind her to contact you if she has any ocular symptoms or questions.
3. Several options should then be presented to DB.
   Option 1. Occlude OD and have her continue to wear present glasses only when reading, using only the distance portions.
   Option 2. Occlude OD and apply press-on –2.00 DS over prescription lens OS.
   Option 3. Prescribe the following as a *temporary* prescription:
   OD: +1.75 –0.50 × 90 = 6 prism diopters base down
   OS: +0.75 DS = 10 prism diopters base in
   OU: +2.00 add
   Option 4. Prescribe progressive addition lens that allows the patient to select the appropriate lens power for the moment, although expensive to fabricate if prism is integrated.

The practitioner should demonstrate and discuss the options with the patient. Choice 1 or 2 is the most likely approach. DB should understand that any lens prescription may become obsolete within a few weeks as the systemic treatment takes effect and the blood sugar stabilizes. Whatever decision she makes, see her in 1 month to verify the lens prescription prior to a more permanent solution.

In virtually all situations, when presented with a significant refractive change because of a variation in the blood sugar, attempt to delay fabricating new spectacles until the underlying condition stabilizes. Patient education and delay in making substantial prescription changes, if at all possible, are essential. In the event prescriptive lens changes cannot be delayed, the patient must understand the fragility of the situation portends the likelihood of this being a temporary lens prescription. If plus spheres are desired, prefabricated "readers" can be useful.

The transitory nature of most findings can be rather dramatic. Gelvin and Thonn report on a patient with resolved cortical cataracts 1 month after the hyperglycemic condition was neutralized.[4]

A less frequent occurrence is represented by patient DC, who has long-standing brittle diabetes with fluctuations in his blood sugar despite compliance in taking insulin. After several visits and verification with his physician, the refractive outcome was two separate pairs of bifocal glasses representing the most frequent powers needed. He enjoys bowling and wishes to see the pins as clearly as possible. He was advised to take both pairs of glasses with him and subjectively decide which gave optimum vision for the bowling pins' distance. This approach works well. Interestingly, DC owns a small retail food shop and usually is able to wear the two prescriptions interchangeably at work. In spite of his reluctance (and the doctor's) to change from something that was working, he too might benefit with a progressive lens when working. His conventional 22-mm-wide flat-top bifocals with low seg heights do not interfere with his bowling style.

Another patient (DD) apparently had untreated diabetes for some time. When she ultimately was treated, she demonstrated a hyperopic refractive shift. Clearly, the change in the blood sugar level can cause a sudden refractive shift in either direction: higher blood sugar usually increases myopia, lower blood sugar more typically increases hyperopia.

Subjective

Case History, Including Signs, Symptoms, and Visual Needs
DD, a 38-year-old woman, noticed a difficulty seeing at near since starting on insulin 2 weeks ago. While she sees well at distance, the computer screen at 25 in. (64 cm) causes strain and reading at 16 in. (40 cm) is difficult unless she moves the book farther away. She previously wore glasses only for distance, but they "don't work anymore." They are 3 years old. There is no other significant history.

Lensometry
OD: −1.25 −0.50 × 180
OS: −1.50 −0.25 × 180

Objective

Ocular Health Assessment
No signs of pathology or abnormality.

Clinical Measures

	At 20 ft (6 m)	At 16 in. (40 cm)
VA (unaided):	OD: 20/20 (6/6)	20/40 (6/12)
	OS: 20/20 (6/6)	20/40 (6/12)
Cover Test:	Sl esop	Sl esop
N.P.C.:	To the nose	
Retinoscopy/	OD: +2.00 −0.25 × 180	
Autorefractor:	OS: +1.75 −0.25 × 180	
Subjective:	OD: +2.00 DS	VA 20/20 (6/6)
	OS: +1.75 −0.25 × 180	VA 20/20 (6/6)
Phoria:	2 Eso	4 Eso
Base-in vergences:	X/5/3	7/8/4
Base-out vergences:	17/18/10	X/18/10
Accom. Amplitude:	4.00 each eye	
Neg. Rel. Accom.:	−2.50	
Pos. Rel. Accom.:	+1.00	

	At 20 ft (6 m)	*At 16 in. (40 cm)*
Fused X-Cyl.:	+1.00 add, 20/20 (6/6)	
Stereo:	25 sec Randot	

Assessment

Hyperopic shift, probably resulting from a reduction in blood sugar. Eyes free of pathology.

Plan

1. Request that DD return at later date and, if no refractive change, prescribe the following:
   OD: +2.00 DS
   OS: +1.75 –0.25 × 180
   OU: +1.00 add
   Glasses are to be worn for computer, reading, and other times as needed.
2. Counsel DD concerning diabetes.
3. Advise DD to return yearly and contact you if she has any visual symptoms before then, to monitor her eye health status and refractive state.

The desirability of a cycloplegic refraction with young patients having diabetes is stressed by Johansen, Sjolie, and Eshoj. They found fewer (12%) apparently myopic patients aged 7–15 with a cycloplegic refraction than the 29% when examined "dry." They recommend a cycloplegic examination on all young patients with diabetes. Since such patients require mydriasis anyway, this should present no major management problem, although it does suggest a change in the more typical process, where a postcycloplegic ("dry") examination strongly influences the results of the "wet" one.[5]

References

1. Records RE. Ocular complications of diabetes mellitus. In: KE Sussman, B Drazin, WE James (eds). *Clinical Guide to Diabetes Mellitus.* New York: Liss, 1987:93–115.

2. *Care of the Patient with Diabetes Mellitus, Optometric Clinical Practice Guideline.* American Optometric Association, St. Louis, 1994:5–8.
3. Cavallerano A. Ocular manifestations of diabetes mellitus. In: JG Classe (ed). *Optometry Clinics,* Vol. 2, No. 2. Norwalk, CT: Appleton and Lange, 1992:93–116.
4. Gelvin JB, Thonn VA. The formation and reversal of acute cataracts in diabetes mellitus. *J Am Optom Assoc.* July 1993;64 (7):471–474.
5. Johansen J, Sjolie AK, Eshoj O. Refraction and retinopathy in diabetic children below 16 years of age. *Acta Ophthalmologica.* December 1994;72(6):674–677.

CHAPTER 11

Refractive Care of the Patient with Cataracts

A significant volume of literature relates to the many aspects of cataracts, including its epidemiology, the lens physiology, surgical correction, and more recently, the comanagement of the surgical patient. Information relevant to these topics is available elsewhere and beyond the scope of this book. An excellent overview and reference list can be found in *Cataract in Adults: Management of Functional Impairment*, published by the U.S. Department of Health and Human Services.[1]

There is no accepted treatment for cataract except removal of the crystalline lens. The enormous impact of cataracts on the public health arena can be illustrated by the fact that an estimated 1.35 million cataract surgeries are performed yearly in the United States, making this the most common surgical procedure on patients over 65.

The emphasis in this chapter is on the refractive implications of the patient with cataracts and their spectacle correction. Modern cataract surgery creates the pseudophakic individual as opposed to the aphakic patient of the past. The patient with an implanted lens requires refractive care, although significantly different in the refractive outcomes than the aphakic patient.

We define *cataracts* generically as crystalline lens opacification that impairs the vision of the patient. The differential diagnosis and quantification of this lens change typically are determined through the use of the biomicroscope, observing the lens through a dilated pupil. In many situations, however, the astute practitioner can function with relative comfort with information and data acquired by other techniques. In learning about the impact of these lens changes on the patient, such basic elements of the encounter as the case history and visual acuity play vital roles.

The refractive care of the patient with cataracts can be subdivided into three subsections: the patient with an incipient cataract, the patient with a maturing cataract, and postsurgical refractive care.

Refraction of the Patient with an Incipient Cataract

It is quite common to encounter some lens changes on patients 60 years old or older. One study reported more than 50% of the patients above 65 years of age had lens opacities, with the percentage increasing with increased age to reach 84% of those 80 or above.[2]

Trevor-Roper and Curran state that, by age 70, over 90% of the population has some evidence of cataract, although many will have negligible visual impairment.[3] The Framingham eye study, using criteria that include a specified reduced level of visual acuity of 20/30 (6/9), found that 15% of the patients between 52 and 85 years of age had cataracts.[4] While the prevalence of cataracts is quite high in all the populations studied, the age of the subjects, the definition of *cataract*, and the method of detection had the vital significance in the numbers found. Regardless of the specific epidemiological numbers, cataracts are relatively common and will increase in frequency as the population ages. Cataracts are typed according to their location within the crystalline lens. Amos reports that nuclear cataracts have approximately twice the frequency of cortical, with posterior subcapsular the least.[5]

For most presurgical patients, the treatment of choice is the correction of the refractive error. The effect of the lens opacification on the patient's life and lifestyle usually determines the wisdom and timing of surgical intervention.

Certain environmental and lifestyle behaviors have been implicated as increasing the risk for these lens changes, including exposure to ultraviolet-B radiation, smoking, alcohol intake, diets low in antioxidants, and specific drugs, such as certain tranquilizers, miotics, and corticosteroids. In addition, trauma and diabetes also may cause cataracts.[6]

As a result, the management plan should include counseling patients accordingly. Managing the patient with an early cataract requires care and sensitivity. Some doctors like to postpone using the term *cataract* until the lens changes affect the patient's vision as consistent with our definition. However, others feel that earlier introduction of the concept is the preferable approach. A term such as *lens changes* serves as a bridge for some practitioners. In any event, do not discuss cataract without a careful explanation of its etiology, physiology, and prognosis as well as the presentation of its surgical correction.

Lens changes may bring about refractive changes, and the clinician should anticipate these possibilities. Nuclear lens changes increase the plus power of the eye and, as a result, are associated with a change in the myopic direction. The refractive change may precede objective verification of the condition.[7] The classic situation of the previously hyperopic individual now not requiring glasses for reading is not necessarily the miracle that the patient perceives (see patient EA). If sufficiently significant in dimension, the clinician can almost predict the existence of this nuclear type of cataract as a result of the case history. Therefore, with nuclear lens changes, the patient's history may indicate visual symptoms suggesting the need for a reduction in the plus (or increase in the minus) power in the spectacle correction. Therefore, the previously myopic patient will indicate the need for stronger minus lenses for distance seeing and less plus in the correction at near, and the previously hyperopic patient will require less plus power for all distances. The presbyopic patient undergoing these lens changes typically reports that the reading correction is "too strong" and reading matter must be held closer to see through the previously effective glasses.

The doctor in considering the most logical reasons for this symptom of glasses being "too strong" in a mature patient should consider the likelihood of nuclear lens changes or diabetes or both. Of additional concern is that the patient with diabetes may develop cataracts at a younger age and these may progress more rapidly than is typical. Therefore, the patient may present with both diabetes and cataracts.[8]

Increased intraocular pressure (IOP; greater than 30 mm Hg) also is a risk factor for cataract progression.[9] While the diagnosis of cataracts requires the observation of the crystalline lens with the biomicroscope, ophthalmoscope, or the retinoscope, the identification of the coexistence of diabetes or elevated IOP requires further investigation starting with the case history. This history dialogue should be programmed to identify the likelihood of diabetes or glaucoma. We need to know if the patient was recently tested for diabetes—how, when, by whom, and the result. A family history of diabetes or glaucoma could be very significant. A patient with diabetes might report symptoms of thirst and frequent urination and may appear obese. We should understand that refractive changes are more rapid with diabetes than with age-related lens changes. An additional clinical confounder is that cataracts caused by hyperglycemia may resolve after the blood sugar normalizes.[10] The response to, "How long have you been aware of these visual changes?" may be particularly revealing. Note that, with these lens changes, the correctable level of vision with spectacles or contact lenses also depends on the entire ocular status, not simply the alteration of the refractive power of the correcting lens. Clearly, a cataract that is sufficiently dense will have an impact on the best-corrected visual acuity, as will coexisting changes in the retina.

We previously discussed the myopic shift observed with nuclear lens changes. Some clinicians also find a shift toward hyperopia with the existence of cortical lens changes. The characteristic appearance of the lens with its peripheral spikes that is best observed through the dilated pupil is a far better diagnostic clue than a hyperopic refractive shift. If the spikes extend closer to or into the pupillary area, they may be observed without dilation or when using the retinoscope.

Another frequently encountered symptom may indicate the likely location of the opacification. The patient who reports seeing better with dim illumination is suggesting the presence of a central lens change. Dim illumination causes an enlarged pupil, which allows rays to circumvent the central opacity. A centrally located opacity diminishes, rather than improves, seeing through a pinhole, so the pinhole acuity is reduced. Theoretically, the patient with cortical lens changes usually prefers high illumination. However, a sufficient number of patients report this preference for high illumination that it is less diagnostic of cortical cataracts.

The posterior subcapsular cataract, as its name implies, is found in the lens cortex just below the capsule, usually in the pupillary area but not necessarily central. It occurs less frequently than the other two, although when located in a critical area it may have significant impact on vision. It is not uncommon to observe a relatively small posterior subcapsular opacity cause diminished acuity. The patient with posterior subcapsular cataracts also may report glare problems, which need to be addressed. These symptoms may be exacerbated when driving in the daytime and facing the sun.[11]

When a posterior subcapsular cataract exists by itself, no characteristic refractive change typically is associated with it.

The refraction of this condition is more a question of understanding the cataract process than altering the process. Additional efforts are necessary when communicating with the patient, both with the case history and the presentation.

The patient, and his or her family, should know what is happening and its prognosis. Future lens changes will alter the "shelf life" of the prescription, with the rapidity of the changes unknown. This patient must be aware that you are available should he or she need you.

Refraction of the Patient with a Maturing Cataract

The patient with a maturing cataract is significantly easier to manage if proper education and counseling took place in the past. Beginning with the onset of the observation of lens changes, it is desirable to illustrate and discuss the physiology and implications of cataracts with the patient at each visit. If this occurred, the earlier dialogue may have prepared the patient for this visit. If, as the result of the examination, a refractive change is contemplated, especially if the acuity improvement is relatively small, it is essential for it to be demonstrated with trial lenses. In spite of the clinician's cautions suggesting limited success, some patients still have the belief that new glasses will achieve the same level of improved vision they experienced in the past. If you are unable to deliver this, it must be carefully demonstrated, so that the patient will understand, and the discussion noted on the patient's record. Having a family member or friend present reinforces this situation.

Subsequent visits by the patient with a history of lens changes and a report of decreased vision stimulates the clinician to expect additional lens changes. The patient may report any of the symptoms listed earlier but to a heightened degree. A sensitive patient may report diminished color perception.[12] The practitioner always should be alert to other conditions that might influence the symptoms. The patient indeed may have the anticipated lenticular changes, something else, or the lens changes combined with something else. For example, the advancing age that increases the risk of progressing cataract formation also increases the risk of such diseases as glaucoma and age-related macular changes. All these conditions may exist in the absence of pain and typically progress slowly. The usual questioning about onset, duration, and progression, while essential, does little to differentiate among these causes of diminished vision in the aging population. Consider other clinical procedures for differential diagnosis.[13]

With the clinical confirmation that the visual loss is caused by lens changes, one viable option at this time is surgery. Prior to recommending surgical intervention, the practitioner needs to know as much as possible about the patient's general health and ocular status as well as the implications of these lens changes on the patient's visual needs. Bilaterally equal cataractous development may allow for fewer options than unilateral development. When one eye is more advanced than the other the patient might weigh the possibility of delay until the vision in the better eye diminishes. The doctor and the patient should consider the wisdom of this, understanding all the parameters. While the principal issue considered is the acuity in the better eye, also be concerned about the effect of the cataract on the patient's binocularity and the importance of this binocularity to the patient. In addition, the refractive situation caused by the lens changes, as well as the patient's health status and lifestyle, enter into the decision-making process. An example of the last issue might be a person with cortical cataracts who drives at night. If this patient wishes to postpone surgery, he or she should be cautioned to reduce or eliminate night driving, since as mentioned earlier, the cortical lens changes tend to reduce the vision with an enlarged pupil. The patient who needs to drive at night might have fewer options in postponing surgery. In general, the clinician functions as a patient advocate particularly with the awareness of the refractive correction no longer addressing the patient's needs. When applied appropriately this gatekeeper role as a patient advocate serves the patient by objectively presenting options and being less influenced by income generation.

Sometimes, the traditional Snellen chart does not adequately quantify the visual problems reported by the patient. In these situations, the practitioner might prefer to use contrast sensitivity measurements. These results may be more consistent with the subjective symptoms reported by the patient. The management options might be more influenced by this test than the Snellen fraction or in addition to the Snellen fraction.[13] However, *Cataract in Adults*[1] cautions that, "the relationship between contrast sensitivity test results and functional impairment has not been adequately studied." Some patients with cataracts, particularly posterior subcapsular cataracts, find that glare is a more disturbing symptom than reduced acuity. The sensitivity to glare can be objectively measured by glare testing instruments. These devices also may prove useful when the postsurgical patient complains of glare.[1]

If the lens opacification is sufficiently dense, the traditional objective measurements of retinoscopy and automated refractors may be less reliable. Increased reliance is placed on the careful subjective examination. The more dense lens may obscure some of the fundus view as well. Other instruments and techniques may be utilized to evaluate the integrity of the eye or its postsurgical visual potential, and they might be employed with patients who contemplate surgery The ethical practitioner presents all the options to the patient, who will be able to make the decision that best suits him or her. While the patient is presented all of the potential options, the clinician may wish to suggest preferences and reasons for them. The patient with cataracts may be emotionally vulnerable; as a result, care and sensitivity should be exercised to assure that all the patient's needs and questions are addressed. These might include details about the surgical procedures, referral options, second opinions, and postsurgical implications. An important element in this presentation is the excellent prognosis both in terms of a low refractive error and the corrected visual acuity, even with high presurgical refractive errors.[14]

Postsurgical Refractive Care

The modern approach to cataract surgery presents far fewer problems than encountered with the aphakic patient of the past. The unilateral aphakic eye invariably eliminated the options of binocularity after correction with either spectacles or contact lenses. The practitioner had the choice of which eye to correct and applied a "balance" lens to the other. The patient with bilateral aphakia typically required unsightly high-powered convex lenses with the attending concerns about spectacle lens thickness, induced prism, and vertex distances. The high plus-powered rigid contact lenses in the past were difficult to fit and sometimes uncomfortable, although an option with some bilateral aphakic patients. While the thrust of this book relates to contemporary refractive care, which would be with the insertion of intraocular lenses (IOLs), those readers faced with the aphakic patient are referred to Milder and Rubin's *The Fine Art of Prescribing Glasses.*[7]

Today's patient with an IOL inserted during the cataract procedure is easier to manage because of the increased likelihood of a refractive outcome of clarity and comfort. When the typically successful outcome ensues, the patient's corrective potential is excellent. The spectacle correction with multifocals or progressive additioned lenses compensates adequately for the absence of accommodation.

If there are no complications, the lenses have sufficient stability for the refractive examination to be performed 1–2 weeks after surgery. The examination of the pseudophakic patient often is quite routine. The basic examination process should include

- *Case History.* This will alert the clinician that a procedure took place. Glare, photophobia, and color distortions may be reported.
- *Health Assessment.* This should include biomicroscopy, ophthalmoscopy, tonometry, plus other tests consistent with symptoms, findings, etc.
- *Objective Refractive Assessment.* This may be difficult due to a poor reflex, which places added emphasis on the subjective examination.
- *Visual Acuity.* VA often is quite good with proper correction.
- *Near Testing.* This may show slightly less than expected add power.
- *Binocular Testing.* Slight misalignment of IOL may result in vertical deviations and/or some anisometropia.[15]

Examples of typical monocular cataract patient problems follow.

Subjective

Case History, Including Signs, Symptoms, and Visual Needs
Patient EA is a 65-year-old woman whose 3-year-old glasses are "too strong," distance seeing is blurred, and she must hold reading too close. She prefers to read at 16 in. (40 cm).

She is in excellent health, according to a recent physical examination.

Lensometry
OD: +1.75 –0.50 × 90
OS: +2.00 –0.50 × 90
OU: +2.50 add

Objective

Ocular Health Assessment
No evidence of ocular disease or abnormalities. Lenses appear clear with biomicroscope.

Clinical Measures

	At 20 ft (6 m)	At 16 in. (40 cm)
VA (with	OD: 20/40 (6/12)	20/40 (6/12)
prescription):	OS: 20/50 (6/15)	20/40 (6/12)
Cover Test:	N/E	N/E
N.P.C.:	N/E	
Retinoscopy/	OD: +1.00 −0.50 × 90	
Autorefractor:	OS: +1.00 −0.50 × 90	
Subjective:	OD: +1.00 −0.50 × 90	VA 20/20 (6/6)
	OS: +1.00 −0.50 × 90	VA 20/20 (6/6)
Phoria:	N/E	
Base-in vergences:	N/E	N/E
Base-out vergences:	N/E	N/E
Accom. Amplitude:	0.50 each eye	
Neg. Rel. Accom.:	N/E	
Pos. Rel. Accom.:	N/E	
Fused X-Cyl.:	+2.50 add, 20/20 (6/6) each eye at	
	16 in. (40 cm)	
Stereo:	N/E	

Assessment

Reduced hyperopic refractive error suggestive of a nuclear lens change in both eyes.

Plan

1. New lens prescription, wear as needed.
2. Monitor crystalline lenses periodically. It is essential in the management of EA to discuss and demonstrate how the new correction will improve the distance vision as well as allow for good vision at 16 in. (40 cm). This would satisfy her presenting symptoms. If she persists in holding reading at 10 in. (25 cm), the previous glasses are better.

We can illustrate a similar situation with a myopic patient. In this example, the myopia appears to progress with symptoms of poor distance and near vision with correction. EA required less plus lens power (or more minus) at both distance and near, as does the myopic patient. The myopic patient requires a correction with higher minus at both far and near. In this situation, the patient also must understand that we are correcting for the desired 16 in. (40 cm) reading distance.

The reason for the careful discussion and demonstration is that we are contradicting **clinical pearl 5**, which states (in part) "be cautious about reducing plus power at near with a presbyopic patient." The operative word here is *cautious* because we have both EA's needs as presented in the history and clinical findings to support this change. Even then we explain and illustrate with lenses the difference between the old and the newer prescriptions. In the event she perceives little or no difference, we would abide by **clinical pearl 5** and make no change.

In the absence of clinical findings of an incipient cataract, some clinicians avoid introducing the concept of a cataract at this time. Others feel that to discuss it now in terms of the prognosis has less emotional baggage and can be "handled" by the patient more easily. Since we define *cataract* as a lens change with an impact on the patient's visual needs, EA's corrected acuity allows the doctor these options.

If the findings presented for EA were the same except with the addition of objective evidence of the lens changes and the refraction resulting in a lower corrected visual acuity, the doctor's communication options are fewer. This patient now meets the objective and subjective criteria for the diagnosis of nuclear cataracts and, quite likely, will carry this diagnosis on all records and insurance forms. This patient should be told about his or her condition, unless there is a very good reason otherwise. If the patient cannot be told, an appropriate surrogate should be informed.

The cataract patient with one eye more advanced than the other, a monocular cataract, may present another dilemma.

Subjective

Case History, Including Signs, Symptoms, and Visual Needs
Patient EB, a 68-year-old man, has a history of bilateral cataracts. This is his first visit to the facility. With glasses, his left eye has poor vision and he sees reasonably well with his right eye but

"could see better." He does not want to consider surgery at this time. He wears his present, 3-year-old glasses constantly. EB prefers to read at 16 in. (40 cm) but his present glasses are best when he holds things closer. EB watches television "across the room" and does some driving, primarily during the daytime. A recent complete physical exam revealed that he is in good health, taking only aspirin.

Lensometry
OD: +4.50 DS
OS: +6.25 DS
OU: +2.50 add

Objective

Ocular Health Assessment
Nuclear cataracts OU, OS more dense. Eyes otherwise healthy.

Clinical Measures

		At 20 ft (6 m)	At 16 in. (40 cm)
VA (with	OD:	20/30 (6/9)	20/30+ (6/9+)
prescription):	OS:	20/80 (6/24)	20/80 (6/24)
Cover Test:		N/E	N/E
N.P.C.:		N/E	
Retinoscopy/	OD:	+4.00 DS	
Autorefractor:	OS:	+5.00 DS	
Subjective:	OD:	+4.00 DS	VA 20/20– (6/6–)
	OS:	+5.00 DS	VA 20/70– (6/21–)
Phoria:		N/E	
Base-in vergences:		N/E	N/E
Base-out vergences:		N/E	N/E
Accom. Amplitude:		0.50 each eye	
Neg. Rel. Accom.:		N/E	
Pos. Rel. Accom.:		N/E	
Fused X-Cyl.:		N/E	
Stereo:		N/E	

Subjectively	OD: With +2.50 add, 20/25 (6/7.5) at 16
Best Near	in. (40 cm)
Acuity:	OS: With +4.00 add, 20/40 (6/12) at 10
	in. (25 cm)

Assessment

Nuclear cataract OS denser than OD. Hyperopia, reduced because of nuclear cataract development.

Plan

1. Monitor lens changes.
2. Order new lens prescription:
   OD +4.00 DS /+2.50 add
   OS +5.00 DS /+2.50 add
3. Educate EB concerning defensive driving with his poor vision OS and why bright daylight may not be optimum for his seeing.
4. Educate about cataracts.

The decision relating to the distance prescription is quite simple. We have a slight visual problem at distance (OD) and can improve on it. Changing the prescription of the OS also improves the vision, although he may not be aware of this unless we demonstrate.

If we were to prescribe for the best acuity at near, we would create the problem of each eye having the best near acuity at a different distance. This may be very bothersome for patients who do not suppress one eye at near; others may adapt to create a type of monovision helping their ranges. The ranges at near for optimum near vision are

OD: 13–16 in. (33–40 cm) with +2.50 add and 0.50 accommodative amplitude

OS: 9–10 in. (23–25 cm) with +4.00 add and 0.50 accommodative amplitude

These are calculated in inches as follows:

OD: Far point of +2.50 lens (add) = 40 in./2.50, or 16 in.
Near point of +3.00 (2.50 add +0.50 amplitude) = 40 in./3.00, or 13 in.

OS: Far point of +4.00 add = 40 in./4.00, or 10 in.
Near point of +4.50 (4.00 add +0.50 amplitude) = 40 in./4.50, or 8.9 in. (or 9 in.)

The solution just indicated is to equalize the near additions to allow EB to have equal accommodative levels in the two eyes at near. When we perform the binocular balance during the distance subjective, by definition we balance the accommodative levels. As a result, equal additions (+2.50 OU in this example) probably will result in similar near ranges for both eyes, which can be measured easily. However, the visual acuity levels are different. The patient *must understand* this. The use of trial lenses helps in the demonstration. The clinician should note this vision discrepancy on the record as well as on the lens prescription form, so that the dispenser can reinforce this concept. EB should be assured that, if it were necessary, the left eye could be improved at near but at the expense of his desired reading distance.

In suggesting this correction we again act contrary to **clinical pearl 5**, do not reduce total plus at near. The patient should be shown how this reduced plus enables his preferred reading distance, reminding him that he reports that, with his current glasses, he needed to hold things closer than he likes. Some clinicians might prescribe +2.75 adds instead of the +2.50, which would compromise the potential problem of acting contrary to **clinical pearl 5**. The decision of +2.50 add and +2.75 add will depend on how EB responds to these lenses in the trial frame. Careful questioning about his reading distance needs also might tilt the scales in one direction or the other. However, if he has any intermediate distance need, the utilization of the +2.50 add as opposed to the +2.75 add will have little effect on this intermediate distance seeing. With the absence of an accommodative amplitude, the patient will have a significant intermediate range of poor vision. With a +2.50 add, the area between approximately 16 in. (40 cm) and clinical infinity is blurred. Prescribing a +1.25 intermediate correction allows for a clear area around 32 in. (81 cm) away from EB. If a traditional trifocal is prescribed, the standard lens has an intermediate power of one half the add. A progressive lens has no such restraint and allows for a range of clear vision approximating from 16 in. (40 cm) to infinity.

EB should understand what is happening to his eyes and the prognosis. Since we did not examine him in the past, we can only guess the extent of the progression in 3 years. We should ask his impression of the rate of progression. That he waited more than 3 years between eye examinations after the diagnosis of cataracts may be significant. The clinician might inquire about this to learn more about the patient. It might be significant, such as fear of surgery, or just time slipping away. We must learn at this visit how he feels about essentially using one eye, if his lifestyle is being affected by his vision. He needs to understand that delay of surgery at this time does not necessarily alter the potential for a successful intervention in the future nor will essentially using one eye at near cause damage to either eye. He should understand that, if other factors intercede, such as a change in health status or another ocular condition, the prognosis in the future may not be similar to today's. This might also be a good time for him to understand modern cataract surgical techniques and their success.

The nonsymmetrical cataract patient may have resulting anisometropia. An example is the patient optimally corrected in each eye by

OD: –3.25 –1.00 × 80   VA 20/20 (6/6)
OS: –6.00 –2.75 × 20   VA 20/80 (6/24)

Some clinicians feel that a difference of >2.00 diopters in the two eyes may cause difficulty with binocularity. Using trial lenses, if the patient suppresses, we might consider a cosmetically balanced OS. This would be noted as follows:

OD: –3.25 –1.00 × 80
OS: –4.00 sph (balance)

If the patient in the optimal correction example reports diplopia with the full prescription, a reduction of spherical and cylindrical power to the left eye may be tried, reducing acuity until the patient comfortably suppresses. However, if the patient is comfortable with the full correction, that can be prescribed. The binocular patient may manifest problems at near, necessitating a slab-off prism to compensate for induced prism at near.

If this patient could be corrected to nearly 20/20 (6/6) OS, one might consider trying contact lenses with full correction. In addition, if that patient is binocular and requires a bifocal correction, we would have to consider prism at near, as discussed in Chapter 7, on anisometropia. Chapter 7 also discusses the asymmetrical cataract patient and the treatment options possible.

References

1. *Cataract in Adults: Management of Functional Impairment*, Clinical Practice Guideline No. 4. Rockville, MD: U.S. Department of Health and Human Services, Public Health Service, Agency for Health Care Policy and Research, February 1993.
2. Sekiryu T, Sakauchi K, Sasaki S, Kato K. Prevalence of lens opacities in ophthalmic screening examination of aged persons. In: O Hockwin, K Sasaki, MC Leske (eds). *Risk Factors for Cataract Development*, Vol. 17. Basel, Switzerland: Karger, 1989:41–46.
3. Trevor-Roper PD, Curran PV. *The Eye and Its Disorders*, 2nd ed. Oxford, England: Blackwell Scientific, 1984:436.
4. Kahn HA, et al. The Framingham eye study. *Am J Epidemiol.* 1977;106:33–41.
5. Amos JF. Optometric care of patients with age-related cataracts. In: JG Classe (ed). *Optometry Clinics*, Vol. 1, No. 2. Norwalk, CT: Appleton and Lange 1991:1–5, 7–8.
6. Ohrloff C. Epidemiology of senile cataract. In: O Hockwin, K Sasaki, MC Leske (eds). *Risk Factors for Cataract Development*, Vol. 17. Basel, Switzerland: Karger, 1989:1–5.
7. Milder B, Rubin ML. *The Fine Art of Prescribing Glasses without Making a Spectacle of Yourself*, 2nd ed. Gainesville, FL: Triad Publishing, 1991:257, 298–309.

8. Cavallerano A. Ocular manifestations of diabetes mellitus. In: JG Classe (ed). *Optometry Clinics.* Norwalk, CT: Appleton and Lange 1992:106.
9. Vesti F. Development of cataract after trabeculectomy. *Acta Ophthal.* December 1933;71(6):777–781.
10. Gelvin JB, Thonn VA. The formation and reversal of acute cataracts in diabetes mellitis. *J Am Optom Assoc.* July 1993 64(7): 471–474.
11. Renier GL. *Clinical Aphakia and Its Spectacle Management.* Chicago: Professional Press, 1997:115.
12. Carter TL. Age-related vision changes: A primary care guide. *Geriatrics.* September 1994;49(9):37–47.
13. Eskridge KJ, Amos JF, Bartlett JD. *Clinical Procedures in Optometry.* Philadelphia: Lippincott, 1991:221–237, 311–320, 436–446.
14. Lyle WA, Jin GJ. Clear lens extraction for the correction of high refractive error. *J Cat Refrac Surg.* May 1993;20(3):273–276.
15. Phillips L, Soltis G. Intraocular lenses and their follow-up in the optometric office. *J Am Optom Assoc.* February 1979;50(2): 149–161.

CHAPTER 12

Refractive Care of the Low-Vision Patient

There are several definitions of *low vision*; and typically when there are several definitions, no one definition satisfies everyone. Some clinicians have defined low vision on the basis of corrected acuity of 20/70 (6/21) or less in the better eye or a visual field of less than 20° or both; Faye considers low vision a bilateral diminished visual acuity or a reduced visual field due to a disorder in the vision system.[1] The resulting decrease in visual performance may be identified by the patient, a government agency, another person, a doctor, an employer, or someone else.[1(p. 1)] An agency, institution, or insurance company is most likely to define it on the basis of a specific visual acuity or visual field loss. For example, the New York state Department of Social Services states its legal definition of low vision as "central visual acuity of 20/60 (6/18) or less in the better eye with best correction" or a specifically identified loss of the visual field. Some practitioners prefer a more-functional approach and define *low vision* as occurring when the corrected vision of the patient with conventional lenses (spectacles or contact lenses) is less than meets the performance needs of that patient. Mehr and Fried specifically define conventional lenses as having additions of +4.00 or less.[2]

In this book, we are concerned primarily with the patient who has limited vision but can be helped with conventional lenses, such as might be found in the usual trial lens set. This typically is the treatment of choice for the near-seeing needs of the low-vision patient and reserves other devices for situations when this more conventional lens approach does not provide suitable vision. The advantages of this approach are that, when it is successful, it affords the low-vision patient the largest field of view, allows the patient to hold reading material in both hands, and the glasses appear "more normal" than a low-vision device. The principal disadvantage of high plus for near is that reading must be held quite close, which in addition to making the patient self-conscious, may block needed light to the reading matter.[3]

The number of patients with a visual impairment will continue to grow as the population ages. These patients will become a larger segment of a primary care practice with time. It is incumbent that the practitioner be willing and able to perform the appropriate services for this population or to refer to competent practitioners who can.[4]

The initial treatment process with the low-vision patient is performing a good refraction. While this appears to be an obvious statement, we all have observed patients identified as having low vision, being amblyopic, or who could have improved function but were victimized by poor refractive technique, analysis, or treatment. The utilization of procedures that may or may not be considered "routine," such as the keratometer, stenopaic slit, retinoscopy at different distances (sometimes referred to as *radical retinoscopy*), and the pinhole and trial lens techniques, may prove highly beneficial. If the patient has reduced vision, care should be taken to create conditions that help to enhance the encounter. The early presentation of test letters that are not visible to the patient sets the stage for failure and increases the tension. We recommend referring to one of the clinical texts relating to low vision care for details on how to perform the examination.[1,5,6]

The typically employed trial set low-vision aid is high plus power for near. This is perfectly consistent with **clinical pearl 13**, reminding us that there is no rule limiting the near add to +2.50 (although some colleagues considered increasing the ceiling to a +3.00 add). The reasons for the +3.00 limit are elusive, but one possible guess is that some laboratories (and those facilities performing their own lab work) do not typically stock finished lenses with higher adds. Another possibility is that higher additions alter the conditions of seeing, such as the reading distance, decentration considerations, and magnification effect, and so are possible areas of confusion. However, in single-vision form or bifocals, high plus for near is an excellent solution for many low-vision patients.

High plus power for near may be employed for the better-seeing eye when the two eyes are sufficiently different or may be prescribed binocularly if the patient is capable of fusing at the appropriate near working distance. Binocular high plus adds typically require base-in prism (or significant decentration) to aid fusion. The amount of prism increases with higher AC/A ratios. In some instances, the fusion can be enhanced with vision therapy. The amount of base-in prism should be the minimal amount required to obtain fusion, equally divided between the two eyes.

When only one eye is corrected, we may employ a "balance" lens of similar appearance (and power) in front of the nonseeing other eye for cosmetic reasons. Some patients may subjectively prefer the nonseeing eye to be occluded. If a specific lens is desired for the other eye to present a separate area of clarity for each eye (monovision), the final decision may hinge on whether cosmesis or convenience is a higher priority, since the appearance of the two will be different. An example of this would be Patient RA.

Subjective

Case History, Including Signs, Symptoms, and Visual Needs

RA is an 86-year-old retiree reporting poor vision for the past 10 years that is getting worse. He has been diagnosed as having cataracts. Since his wife was blind after cataract surgery, he rejects that approach unless the surgeon can guarantee that he will see better after surgery. His present glasses are 3 years old, "okay" for television when he sits close, but poor for reading even with his hand magnifier, which he does not like. He has no other significant ocular history. His medical status is "fair," with a long history of heart problems, for which he takes medications.

Lensometry

OD: −3.00 DS
OS: −3.00 DS (balance lens)
OU: +3.00 add

Objective

Ocular Health Assessment

Bilateral cataracts OD, OS. Dilated fundus examination reveals no other abnormality or pathology.

Clinical Measures

		At 20 ft (6 m)	*At 13 in. (33 cm)*
VA (with	OD:	20/80 (6/24)	20/100 (6/30)
prescription):	OS:	20/400 (6/120)	20/400 (6/120)
Cover Test:		LXT	LXT'
N.P.C.:		N/E	
Retinoscopy/	OD:	Approx. –3.00	
Autorefractor:	OS:	Approx. plano	
Subjective:	OD:	–3.00 DS	VA 20/80 (6/24)
	OS:	+1.00 DS	VA 20/400 (6/120)
Phoria:		N/E	N/E
Base-in vergences:		N/E	N/E
Base-out vergences:		N/E	N/E
Accom. Amplitude:		N/E	
Neg. Rel. Accom.:		N/E	
Pos. Rel. Accom.:		N/E	
Fused X-Cyl.:		N/E	
Stereo:		No fusion	
Other Near Testing:		+5.00 add OD gives best near acuity at 8 in. (20 cm)	

Assessment

Reduced vision due to bilateral cataracts, OS much worse than OD.

Plan

1. Discuss cataracts and modern surgical techniques—but do not guarantee success.
2. The patient should be presented with a spectacle treatment plan:
   OD: –3.00 DS (giving best distance acuity)
   OS: –3.00 DS (balance lens)
   for distance only.

OD: +2.00 DS
OS: +2.00 DS (balance)
for near only. The patient uses the right eye for distance and near. A variation of this would be OU −3.00 DS/+5.00 add.

In making the presentation (and prior to prescribing), it is a good idea to demonstrate to the patient how it is necessary to function (the distances required) and what the spectacles will look like. Patients with poor vision often are quite sensitive about appearing different, so it is essential that they are aware of these aspects of their tentative correction. The total absence of fusion would allow for this approach.

3. Have patient return in 1 year to monitor progression of the cataracts.

With other patients, if binocular high plus for near is contemplated because of similar lens powers, acuities, and strong fusional capabilities, the new near close working/distance can create a disruption in the binocularity of the patient. The compensating prismatic needs of the patient may be accomplished by centering the high plus lenses nasally, providing base-in prism. Some authorities suggest that a practical ceiling is a +10.00 DS addition, which has a working distance of approximately 4 in. To prescribe anything higher is a somewhat futile attempt to compensate for the convergence demand.[7] For high adds with binocularity, the following calculation can be applied.

Assuming, for this calculation, a distance pupillary measure (PD) of 64 mm, a +10.00 DS addition, and an average distance of 27 mm from the center of rotation of the eye to the back surface of the spectacles,

$$\text{Decentration} = \frac{27 \text{ mm} \times (\text{PD})}{\text{Lens working distance} + 27}$$

The focal distance of a +10.00 add is 100 mm; therefore,

$$\text{Decentration} = \frac{27 \times 64}{100 + 27} = \frac{1728}{127} = 14 \text{ mm}$$

Total decentration = Decenter in 14 mm from
the optical center (or 7 mm in, for each lens)

Another method that could be used is to simply measure the interpupillary distance for the appropriate working distance. If the patient is to see at 8 in. (20 cm), measure the near centration distance from 8 in. (20 cm) away.

Cole reports that a +4.00 DS lens addition might serve the intermediate distance needs of the low-vision patient whose near add is greater than +4.00.[8] In these situations, he considers a range of 8–13 in. as intermediate, since it helps the patient with such tasks as writing and eating. The true range of the patient often defies the 10-in. calculated far-point range expected with a +4.00 lens. He recommends a simplified "test" process, in which he has the patient observe his or her hand at 8–10 in. He then places +4.00 trial lenses over the patient's distance prescription and asks if the lenses make things better. If so, he may modify the +4.00 power and prescribe it for specific tasks The patient must understand the limitations of this intermediate prescription. It is not for reading or television, or what traditionally was an intermediate distance.[8,9,10]

Since the entire low-vision exam is best carried out with trial lenses and a trial frame, the near testing is easily sequenced, starting with the foundation of the best distance prescription found. Allowing the patient to hold materials that he or she wishes to see, start with a likely lens, then modify it. The patient should demonstrate improved vision to justify increasing power. When the best vision at the best possible distance is determined, verify whether reducing the near prescription by 0.50 or 1.00 diopter reduces the vision. Since higher plus decreases the working distance, lower powers are desirable because they allow the patient to move the near material farther away. During this phase of the exam, the patient must be instructed to hold the near materials at the distance determined by the lenses, where vision should be best. The balanced need of improved vision and maximum working distance should become quite apparent. Modifications are made based on these combined needs of the near working preferences with the lens requirements. Although ranges can be calculated, they should be demonstrated using trial lenses. These ranges may vary from the theoretical, and this trial technique allows the doctor and the patient to appreciate the advantages and limitations of the tentative lens prescription.

Several methods may be used to predict the reading add (and corresponding near magnification power) from the patient's visual acuity. This predicted add is a starting point and must be modified utilizing trial lenses. The modification usually attempts to balance the magnification with the working distance needed by the patient. The Lighthouse has a chart that converts the Snellen near acuity into the tentative lens power needed to read 1 M–size print (20/50 equivalent) at 16 in. (40 cm) (Table 12-1).

Add (Diopters) for 1 M Print

The chart in Table 12-1 provides a starting point that needs to be tested and modified using trial lenses. Note that the focal distance of a +10.00 diopter lens is 4 in. (10 cm). The +10.00 lens will *not* allow the patient needing to see 1 M (20/50) equivalent acuity at near at the 16 in. (40 cm) testing distance. The chart allows the practitioner to convert the near acuity when measured at 8 or 16 in. (20 to 40 cm) to a tentative near addition.

Table 12-1 Measured Snellen Near Equivalent

Letter Size	Acuity at 16 in. (40 cm)	Add in Diopters for 1.0 M Print
8.0 M	20/400 (6/120)	20 DS
6.4 M	20/300 (6/90)	15 DS
5.0 M	20/250 (6/75)	12 DS
4.0 M	20/200 (6/60)	10 DS
	At 8 in. (20 cm)	
8.0 M	20/800	40 DS
6.4 M	20/600	30 DS
5.0 M	20/500	25 DS
4.0 M	20/400	20 DS

Source: Reprinted with permission from The Lighthouse. Near Vision Acuity Chart LH-NV-5. New York: The Lighthouse.

Another method is to use the following formula:

$$\text{Predicted add} = \frac{\text{Distance Snellen denominator}}{\text{Near desired Snellen denominator}} \times 2.50$$

(the 2.50 is referenced to 16 in., or 40 cm).

For example, the patient measures 20/400 (6/120) at distance and needs 20/50 (6/15) equivalent near acuity (1 M print). The examiner should start with a +20.00 DS addition and present materials that the patient wishes to see—newspapers, sewing— encouraging the patient to hold the material at approximately 2 in. (5 cm), then subjectively modify both the lens power and the working distance. The use of real-life materials is important, since our reading card has better contrast and spacing than most objects that the patient wishes to see.

A third method of estimating the tentative near add is to use the reciprocal of the distance acuity as an add that allows a patient to read 1 M–size print. Therefore, if the patient's distance acuity is 20/200 (6/60), we can calculate

200/20 = 10; therefore, start with a +10.00 OS add. (The working distance of this +10.00 add would be 4 in. [10 cm].)[11]

Any of these methods is appropriate.[12]

RB is an interesting patient.

Subjective

Case History, Including Signs, Symptoms, and Visual Needs
RB is a 78-year-old man with a history of age-related macular degeneration (ARMD), OD much worse than OS. He wants to read newspapers and menus. He uses a telescope for viewing television but wants conventional looking glasses for reading in public. His present glasses are unsatisfactory.

Lensometer
OD: +3.25 DS
OS: +2.50 –1.50 × 90
OU: +3.00 add

Objective

Ocular Health Assessment

ARMD OU, incipient cataracts OU.

Clinical Measures

	At 20 ft (6 m)	At 16 in. (40 cm)
VA (corrected):	OD: <20/400 (<6/120)	<20/400 (<6/120)
	OS: 20/150 (6/45)	20/150 (6/45)
Pinhole:	OD: <20/400 (<6/120)	
	OS: 20/150 (6/45)	
Cover Test:	N/E	N/E
N.P.C.:	N/E	
Retinoscopy/	OD: +3.00 DS	
Autorefractor:	OS: +2.50 DS	
Subjective:	OD: +3.00 DS	VA N/E
	OS: +2.50 DS	VA 20/150 (6/45)
Phoria:	N/E	N/E
Base-in vergences:	N/E	N/E
Base-out vergences:	N/E	N/E
Accom. Amplitude:	N/E	
Neg. Rel. Accom.:	N/E	
Pos. Rel. Accom.:	N/E	
Fused X-Cyl.:	N/E	
Stereo:	N/E	

Referring to the Lighthouse chart a near equivalent acuity of 20/150 (6/45) requires an +8.00 diopter addition to see 1 M-size print at 5 in. (12.5 cm). With this patient reading a newspaper, the best compromise between reading distance and acuity is found with a +8.50 DS add.

Assessment

Reduced acuity due to ARMD and cataracts, OD poorer than OS.

Plan

1. New near prescription in a half-eye frame:
   OD: +9.00 DS (balance)
   OS: +11.00 DS

Polycarbonate lenses (to protect better-vision eye) designed to be as thin as possible.
2. Monitor eye health.
3. Educate RB concerning possible prognosis.
4. Educate RB on apparent relationship of lifestyle changes (smoking, diet, dietary supplements) to ARMD.

In establishing the criteria for this chapter, we said that we would discuss those low-vision situations that may be helped with lenses found in the trial set. At times, prisms may be utilized with low-vision patients for other than binocular fusion. One example of this is with a patient having nystagmus. A yoked prism may be used to redirect the image toward the null point. Prisms also may be appropriate in other situations, caused by trauma or disease. We feel that a detailed discussion of this topic is beyond the scope of this book and suggest seeking information from the low-vision or rehabilitative literature before proceeding.

Other situations that may or may not meet the various criteria for low vision also are in the realm of basic refractive care. One example of this is the patient with a high refractive error who may demonstrate better vision with contact lenses. The examiner should keep this possibility in mind when managing a patient with a high error. If the patient reports that contact lenses did not provide the desired improvement in the past, learn more about the previous experience, since improvement might be possible with a different contact lens material or design. Improvement also may be derived from spectacle lenses of different materials or design. Aspheric surfaces with prescriptions of greater than +8.00, along with reduced center and edge thickness and a reasonably flat posterior surface, sometimes result in better vision and, in addition, cosmetically more desirable spectacles.[6]

Acknowledgment

We thank Dr. Roy Cole for his help with this chapter.

References

1. Faye EE. *Clinical Low Vision*, 2nd ed. Boston: Little, Brown, 1984:3–55.
2. Mehr EB, Fried AN. *Low Vision Care*. Chicago: Professional Press, 1975:1.
3. Cole RG. Considerations in low vision prescribing. *Problems in Optometry*. September 1991;3(3):416–432.
4. Raasch TW, Leat SJ, Kleinstein RN, Bullimore MA, Cutter GR. Evaluating the value of low-vision services. *J Am Optom Assoc*. May 1997;68(5):287–295.
5. Bailey IL. Low vision visual acuity. In: JB Eskridge, JF Amos, JD Bartlett (eds). *Clinical Procedures in Optometry*. Philadelphia: Lippincott, 1991:754–761.
6. Nowakowski RW. *Primary Low Vision Care*. Norwalk, CT: Appleton and Lange, 1994:21–53, 131–132.
7. Weiss NJ, Brown WL. Use of prism in low vision. In: SA Cotter (ed). *Clinical Use of Prism*. St. Louis: Mosby, 1995:294–297.
8. Cole RG. Clinical insights . . . the 4 diopter intermediate. *J Vis Rehab*. 1992;6(4):13–14.
9. Rosenthal BP, Cole RG. *Functional Assessment of Low Vision*. St. Louis: Mosby, 1996:27–44.
10. Bennett AG, Rabbetts RB. *Clinical Visual Optics*, 2nd ed. Boston: Butterworth–Heinemann, 1989:303, 304.
11. Brown WL. Low vision. In: KL Alexander (ed). *Primary Eye Care*. Philadelphia: Lippincott, 1995:499–538.
12. Elam JH. Analysis of methods for predicting near-magnification power. *J Am Optom Assoc*. January 1997;68(1):31–36.

CHAPTER 13

The Dissatisfied Patient

All practitioners of health care encounter dissatisfied patients. It is estimated that approximately 7% of the patients of private practitioners, optometrists, and ophthalmologists had to return with their glasses because of some degree of dissatisfaction.[1] Our experience as practitioners and supervisors estimates a lower level, approximately 3–3.5%. Whatever the number, everyone experiences some unhappy patients. The complete absence of complaints is unrealistic. Rather than suggest that this doctor is perfect, it indicates that, for whatever reason, the unhappy patient has gone elsewhere. To suggest that all dissatisfied patients are the doctor's fault also is inaccurate. However, after many years of caring for and reviewing the records of unhappy patients, it is apparent that many of these returning encounters could have been prevented in either the examination room or the dispensary. The objective review of the causes of dissatisfaction and their resolution is a valuable lesson in patient care. A goal for all practitioners is to reduce the number of disgruntled patients, if for no other reason than its negative impact on our egos and pocketbooks. In addition, since clinicians are concerned with preventive care, the object in presenting this selection of situations is to focus on how they might have been averted. Unhappy patients are less likely to retain their confidence in the doctor, which may result in lessened compliance, potentially diminishing the outcome of the care rendered. Dissatisfied patients may actively deter other patients from seeking care. Our goal is to sensitize the reader to those situations that more frequently generate dissatisfaction. Prudent care can reduce the number of dissatisfied

291

patients, although also be aware that some patients will not be satisfied by some doctors; some may not be satisfied by any doctor. We observed patients who return with a "problem" every time they receive care. However, if one takes the attitude that the patient is the problem, successful resolution will not happen. Analysis with an open mind allows for some of our best lessons to come from apparently unanticipated outcomes. Greet this situation with the positive feeling that the patient still has sufficient confidence to allow you to resolve the problem.

In conceptualizing this text, we consider that the examination must be customized to meet the needs of the specific patient. When working with dissatisfied patients, this is particularly true. Since the patient recently has had a complete examination, the doctor should now be specifically oriented to the presenting problem. If, however, there is a suspicion that a procedure should be repeated or another performed, the sophisticated practitioner will function accordingly. In most cases, the only tests warranted are those to identify and verify the problem(s) and work toward a solution. **Clinical pearl 1**, "Listen to your patient," is particularly vital with the returning patient. The complaining patient may suggest the solution to the problem. We have observed patients who learned how to position their spectacles to resolve their problem, most often taking advantage of lens effectivity, but we also observed that a few patients rotate their lenses indicating a cylindrical axis problem.

The most typical aspect of problem cases is that they seldom are complex. In fact, a combination of some of the clinical pearls of conventional wisdom with good communication and demonstration techniques goes far in preventing or resolving most of the presenting problems. Since some of the best lessons are learned from mistakes, we provide the opportunity to learn from others' errors, miscalculations, and misjudgments.

Although this is not a book on communication techniques, the unhappy, sometimes irate, returning patient also needs the appropriate responses to regain confidence.

Most of our experiences primarily were not due to poor technique, although at times inaccurate findings can be responsible for problems. In a teaching institution, some of the grief patients feel does stem from this cause, but interestingly, these are in the minority. One of the more common examples in this category is when poor lensometry is the initial culprit. If in doubt, recheck the lensometry, particularly if someone else performed the measurement. Never assume that the lenses were fabricated correctly.

For a short period of time, one of us kept a log of the cause-for-grief patients to get a sense of frequencies. During that period the following predominated:

1. Reduction of overall plus for near when compared to previous glasses.
2. New, stronger bifocal addition changed the range of clear vision and reduced vision for the computer.
3. Space distortion with new glasses.
4. Patient not understanding the limitations of the new glasses.
5. New stronger minus lenses were identified as "too strong." (One of the buzz words that attracts potential grief is for the doctor to use the word *stronger* in describing a lens change, particularly with myopic patients who have a history of stronger and stronger lenses accompanied by diminishing unaided acuity.)
6. New lenses prescribed for asymptomatic patient who now reports that the old ones were better.

As mentioned earlier, prevention is the goal. Therefore, it is important to keep in mind the appropriate pearls, particularly **clinical pearl 18**, "Remind all patients that they may have to adapt to their new glasses" (even when the prescription is identical or virtually identical to previous glasses).

All patients should be advised that they should contact the office if they have any questions or concerns. The message here is that you provide continuing care and are accessible. This approach also allows the office to triage the patient as needed.

A significant group of dissatisfied patients stems from problems best resolved in the dispensary. Sometimes, the verbalized complaint is merely a camouflage to hide unhappiness with the appearance or physical comfort of the spectacles or the decision of whether or not to have multifocals (and what type). It is sufficiently common for a patient to complain about clarity or visual comfort when, in reality, he or she has another agenda. A typical example is the situation of AA.

Subjective

Case History, Including Signs, Symptoms, and Visual Needs
AA is a 33-year-old woman who returns 2 weeks after receiving new glasses with the following complaints: Vision with the new glasses is "too intense" and the frame received was not the one ordered.

Lensometry
OU: –7.75 DS

Previous prescription was OU –7.50 DS, with 20/20 (6/6) acuity and no symptoms.

Clinical Measures

	At 20 ft (6 m)	At 16 in. (40 cm)
VA (with	OD: 20/20 (6/6)	20/20 (6/6)
prescription):	OS: 20/20 (6/6)	20/20 (6/6)
Cover Test:	N/E	N/E
N.P.C.:	N/E	
Retinoscopy/	OD: –7.75 DS	
Autorefractor:	OS: –7.75 DS	
Subjective:	OD: –7.75 DS	VA 20/20 (6/6)
	OS: –7.75 DS	VA 20/20 (6/6)
Phoria:	N/E	N/E
Base-in vergences:	N/E	N/E
Base-out vergences:	N/E	N/E
Accom. Amplitude:	N/E	
Neg. Rel. Accom.:	N/E	
Pos. Rel. Accom.:	N/E	
Fused X-Cyl.:	N/E	
Stereo:	N/E	

Assessment

Myopia OU with very slight increase in each eye.

Plan

1. Reorder new lenses with previous lens prescription of –7.50 OU fabricated with similar materials and lens curves as "old" glasses.
2. Investigate whether the frame order was inaccurate.
3. Counsel AA concerning the effects of lens changes and the likely future scenario.

In this situation, new lenses of –7.50 DS (duplicating her previous prescription) were ordered in a different frame.

Many myopic patients fear that stronger lenses lead to myopic progression. Was it the lens change, the frame, or both, that motivated AA to return? We will never know. The clinician needs to be alert to the possibility of the patient having a hidden agenda. Perhaps, when the initial doctor discussed the possible lens change, AA's reaction would have been revealing. Indicating that the new lens was a bit stronger and then demonstrating the slight acuity difference may have elicited a reaction on the part of the patient that would have predicted the outcome. (The patient's belief that the frames were changed may have been sufficient to motivate the return; if so, the dispenser might have resolved the issue.)

A commonly encountered problem is illustrated by Patient AB. In this situation, prescribing a stronger lens prescription at near diminished the patient's clarity for the computer screen at 25 in. (64 cm). He had been using the previous glasses with a weaker addition for this intermediate distance and reading. The location of the computer screen allowed this without him stretching his neck. His accommodative amplitude was insufficient to compensate when he tried to use the distance portion of the bifocals and the reduced distance range through the new addition was too close for the computer screen. His intermediate range of clear vision was deficient with his new bifocal glasses. The following are data from AB's return visit.

Subjective

Case History, Including Signs, Symptoms, and Visual Needs

AB is a 64-year-old banker who originally complained of diminished vision at 16 in. (40 cm) with his 2-year-old bifocal lens prescription. His distance seeing was "OK" with his glasses and when using his bifocal, and leaning forward a bit, the computer also was "OK." The previous prescription was OU +2.00 DS/+2.00 add. He habitually reads at 16 in. (40 cm) and the computer screen is at 25 in. (64 cm). His most recent examination, 3 weeks ago, resulted in OU +2.00 DS/+2.50 add. He returns with this prescription, saying that his reading is clearer but with a complaint of poor vision for the computer screen.

Objective

Ocular Health Assessment
N/E

Clinical Measures

	At 20 ft (6 m)	At 16 in. (40 cm)
VA (with new prescription):	OD: 20/20 (6/6)	20/20 (6/6)
	OS: 20/20 (6/6)	20/20 (6/6)
Cover Test:	N/E	N/E
N.P.C.:	N/E	
Retinoscopy/	OD: +2.00 DS	
Autorefractor:	OS: +2.00 DS	
Subjective:	OD: +2.00 DS	VA 20/20 (6/6)
	OS: +2.00 DS	each eye
Phoria:		
Base-in vergences:		
Base-out vergences:		
Accom. Amplitude:	0.50	
Neg. Rel. Accom.:	N/E	
Pos. Rel. Accom.:	N/E	
Fused X-Cyl.:	+2.50 Add resulting in 20/20 VA in each eye at 16 in. (40 cm)	
Stereo:	N/E	

Measured Ranges of Clarity for Each Eye with Bifocal Correction:
Distance: 60 in. (150 cm) to infinity
Near: 16 in. (40 cm) to 13 in. (33 cm)

There is an area of poor vision between 60 in. (150 cm) and 16 in. (40 cm) that includes the distance to the computer screen. If a trifocal is prescribed with a typical intermediate power of one half the add, or +1.25 in this case, the range through the intermediate is 32 in. (81 cm) to 23 in. (58 cm). This would provide clarity at distance, near, and the intermediate computer distance. The situation also can be resolved by prescribing a progressive lens allowing the patient to, in effect, select the necessary power. This also gives the patient the flexibility of utilizing another computer, which may be placed slightly differently.

Assessment

Intermediate clarity through the new bifocals.

Plan

Prescribe the equilivant of a +1.25 add for the computer. This may be in the form of trifocals, occupational glasses, or progressive multifocals. If occupational bifocals are prescribed its form could be OU +3.25 DS/+1.25 add. This would provide AB clear vision for the computer screen when using the top portion of the bifocals and a total of +4.50 through the bifocal segment for reading hard copy. The patient should understand that these glasses are designed for the computer, and he should not attempt to use them for distance seeing, as the vision will be blurred. It would be desirable to demonstrate the advantages and disadvantages of these with trial lenses.

Another approach would be a trifocal with the following:

OU: +2.00 DS/+1.25 intermediate/+2.50 add

Other occupational lens designs may be selected, if appropriate or as they become available. The options with their pros and cons should be discussed with AB and a joint decision made.

The reason AB returned was his complaint that, although he saw better for reading (at 16 in., 40 cm) with his new glasses, the computer screen (at 25 in., 64 cm) was not as clear as with his previous glasses. The measured and calculated ranges of clear vision verified the symptoms.

If the patient must have clear vision at 16 in. (40 cm) and 25 in. (64 cm), the clinician should measure and verify the acuity at these distances on the near-point rod utilizing appropriately sized material. Simulating these conditions helps assure the accuracy of the patient's needs.

Patient AB illustrates **clinical pearl 11**, "Never prescribe without understanding the patient's visual needs (and distances) and appreciating the effect of the new prescription(s) on these needs (and distances)." These needs should be identified during the case history and noted on the patient's record.

A variation of this occurs when the clinician does not learn the patient's visual habits and needs or fails to give them the attention required. The distance and position of viewing matter, as well as ergonomic factors such as lighting, reflections, and shadows, help in customizing solutions. The examiner should be knowledgeable and prepared to offer recommendations relating to these problems.

A different type of problem is illustrated by Patient AC, who returns with the complaint of difficulty reading through the new glasses. She reports that her previous glasses were better at near. Additional questioning reveals that she sometimes uses the glasses for near as well as distance, even though they were prescribed "for distance only." The patient's return results in a breakdown of communication. The clinician assumes that the patient wears the glasses as prescribed, an assumption that proves inaccurate. A good way to specify when distance glasses are to be worn is to tell the patient the material to be seen through the distance lenses must be beyond arm's length. This will help the patient who reports that he or she cannot read road signs with the reading glasses. The results from the recheck examination are as follows.

Subjective

Case History, Including Signs, Symptoms, and Visual Needs

AC, a 38-year-old bus driver, initially presented with no symptoms other than complaints of flashing of lights. At this time, she again reports these flashes but now is not seeing as well for near as with her previous glasses. She reported no other ocular or visual symptoms. Her previous prescription, 1 year old, is for distance only:

OD: –1.75 DS   VA 20/30 (6/9)
OS: –1.75 –0.25 × 90   VA 20/30 (6/9)

Her most recent prescription is

OD: –2.25 DS
OS: –2.25 –0.25 × 90

Lensometry
Prescription correct as ordered.

Objective

Ocular Health Assessment
No ophthalmoscopic findings explain the flashes of light.

Clinical Measures

	At 20 ft (6 m)	*At 16 in. (40 cm)*
VA (with latest	OD: 20/20 (6/6)	20/20 (6/6)
prescription):	OS: 20/20 (6/6)	20/20 (6/6)
Cover Test:	N/E	N/E
N.P.C.:	N/E	
Retinoscopy/	OD: –2.50 DS	VA 20/20 (6/6)
Autorefractor:	OS: –2.50 –0.25 × 90	VA 20/20 (6/6)
Subjective:	OD: –2.25 DS	VA 20/20 (6/6)
	OS: –2.25 –0.25 × 90	VA 20/20 (6/6)

	At 20 ft (6 m)	At 16 in. (40 cm)
Phoria:	N/E	N/E
Base-in vergences:	N/E	N/E
Base-out vergences:	N/E	N/E
Accom. Amplitude:	5.50 each eye	
Neg. Rel. Accom.:	2.50	
Pos. Rel. Accom.:	1.50	
Fused X-Cyl.:	+0.75, orthophoria laterally with this tentative add	
Stereo:	N/E	

Assessment

As with her previous visit, no cause for flashes is observed. The amount of myopia found is similar to that recently prescribed and higher than the entering glasses. Subjectively, she perceives diminished near acuity, although findings do not support this.

Plan

Discuss the situation with the patient, demonstrate the acuity issues, and consider one of two plans:

1. Suggest using the new prescription for driving, particularly at night.
2. Suggest continuing to use the previous prescription for distance seeing other than driving, such as television or walking around.

Educate AC by demonstrating the differences in seeing with the various glasses, including implications for the future. She should understand that near seeing probably will be additionally compromised through any lenses designed primarily for distance vision, more so in the future as her eyes change with time. This may be a good time to discuss presbyopia.

Regarding the reported flashes of light, since we see no cause, a decision should be made whether to recommend having another person perform a dilated fundus examination at this time.

At the very least, she needs to be aware of the need to contact us if they continue.

If we believes the patient will benefit from better distance vision, the risks and benefits must be carefully stated and demonstrated. A valid argument could be made that the added acuity could be beneficial to a bus driver, particularly at night. In addition, with 5.50 diopters of accommodative amplitude, we might guess that she would see sufficiently well at near with the new correction, in spite of her initial subjective awareness. In this situation, although the patient is apparently asymptomatic regarding distance acuity, a change in the prescription should be considered. This is a difficult call, one that can be defended either by initially changing nothing or suggesting increased minus. However, if the patient is advised that better distance vision might be initially accompanied with an apparent near problem and this is demonstrated, acceptance of the stronger prescription would be enhanced.

Some patients defy a simple solution, such as AD. Pertinent findings from his reexamination follow.

Subjective

Case History, Including Signs, Symptoms, and Visual Needs

AD is a 30-year-old artist, with slightly blurred distance vision and some asthenopia associated with prolonged work without glasses. He paints primarily at arm's length, while viewing a model at 15 ft. With his new glasses, vision is clear but distorted. He originally stated that he never injured his eyes or wore glasses. The lenses prescribed were

OD: Plano -1.00×75
OS: Plano -1.00×105

Objective

Ocular Health Assessment
N/E

Clinical Measures

	At 20 ft (6 m)	At 16 in. (40 cm)
VA (no	OD: 20/30 (6/9)	20/20 (6/6)
prescription):	OS: 20/30 (6/9)	20/20 (6/6)
VA (new	OD: 20/20 (6/6)	20/20 (6/6)
prescription):	OS: 20/20 (6/6)	20/20 (6/6)
Cover Test:	Ortho	Ortho
N.P.C.:	N/E	
Retinoscopy/	OD: +0.25 −1.00 × 75	
Autorefractor:	OS: Plano −1.00 × 105	
Subjective:	OD: Plano −1.00 × 75	VA 20/20 (6/6)
	OS: Plano −1.00 × 105	VA 20/20 (6/6)
Phoria:	N/E	N/E
Base-in vergences:	N/E	N/E
Base-out vergences:	N/E	N/E
Accom. Amplitude:	N/E	
Neg. Rel. Accom.:	N/E	
Pos. Rel. Accom.:	N/E	
Fused X-Cyl.:	Plano	
Stereo:	30 sec. arc (Titmus)	

Placing this tentative prescription in a trial frame and having the patient view the room caused space distortion that was eliminated by rotating toward axis 90° in each eye. However, while the distortion was eliminated, the acuity was reduced.

Assessment

Simple myopic oblique astigmatism verified.

Plan

1. No change in spectacle prescription found.
2. We discuss the reasons for the space distortion with AD and the advantages and disadvantages of this or a modified prescription (with axis 85 OD and 95 OS).
3. We discuss the possibility of contact lenses.

AD then reports a similar experience 6 months ago with another doctor. When he presents these glasses, they are identical to the lenses originally prescribed.

AD is advised that the ultimate likelihood of good vision and reduced ocular discomfort depends on him adjusting to the astigma-reducing glasses. His trained eye probably exacerbates the subjective visual distortion. Rather than exert the effort, he came to this clinic, probably seeking a second opinion. This illustrates **clinical pearl 15**, concerning the wisdom of the previous doctor.

An appropriate doctor/patient relationship is based on truth, and if either party deceives the other, this diminishes the contract. Here, AD withheld important information. In spite of this, we must help AD, who is given several treatment alternatives:

1. He can continue to attempt to adjust to the glasses. Additional time and effort might succeed. (We could not know whether he gave it any effort in the past.) He is urged to try the glasses for all visual tasks for 2 weeks. The more he wears them, the greater is the chance of success. If successful, this option has the best potential to provide clear, comfortable vision. AD responds positively to the concept of a finite period of time required to attempt to adjust, as opposed to an open-ended period he previously received. Experientially, we find that, if an honest attempt is made and no improvement shown in 2 weeks, adjustment may not happen.

2. He is advised that another approach to achieve clarity and comfort without distortion might be with contact lenses. He rejects this approach.

3. Yet another alternative is a spectacle correction with the prescription at axis 90 in each eye. This is presented as a "modified" prescription, to be worn for several weeks, at which time the situation again will be monitored. When the lenses are inserted in a trial frame, the space distortion is eliminated. The patient is advised that, although the likelihood of the space distortion is significantly lessened, his vision would be slightly poorer and the outcome concerning a reduction in asthenopia is unknown and would be learned retrospectively,

after he wears the new prescription. The effect of lens rotation on clarity and space distortion could be demonstrated.

Interestingly, the patient chooses to attempt to adjust to the original cylindrical prescription. Although the patient is advised to telephone and report on his progress, he neither telephones nor returns. Therefore, we have no way of assessing the outcome of the encounter. The utilization of **clinical pearl 4**, "Use trial lenses in a trial frame with every significant lens change," would have anticipated the space distortion and possibly prevented the subsequent visits. No clinical pearl relates to the patient withholding important information from the examiner.

Patient AE had a different problem, one that is not very uncommon among dissatisfied patients. The original doctor delivered improved vision with her new glasses, but the patient either anticipated, or hoped for, more than could be delivered. The important information from the encounter follows.

Subjective

Case History, Including Signs, Symptoms, and Visual Needs

AE is a 78-year-old woman who originally complained of poor vision with her 2-year-old glasses and finds seeing not much better with the new ones. AE has a history of cataracts but fears surgery because of her "weak heart." She takes no heart medication but uses dietary supplements under the supervision of a "nutritionalist." With her permission, we contact her physician, who reports that AE is in good health and takes no medications.

Lensometry

New glasses,

OD: $+3.00 -1.00 \times 90$
OS: $+3.25 -1.25 \times 90$
    $+2.50$ add

Previous glasses,

OD: +2.25 –1.00 × 90   VA 20/40 (6/12)
OS: +2.75 –1.25 × 90   VA 20/40 (6/12)
OU: +2.50 add

Objective

Ocular Health Assessment
Cataracts OU verified.

Clinical Measures

	At 20 ft (6 m)	*At 16 in. (40 cm)*
VA (with new	OD: 20/30+ (6/9+)	20/30 (6/9)
prescription):	OS: 20/25– (6/7.5–)	20/30 (6/9)
Cover Test:	N/E	N/E
N.P.C.:	N/E	
Retinoscopy/	OD: +3.00 –1.00 × 90	
Autorefractor:	OS: +3.25 –1.25 × 90	
Subjective:	OD: +3.00 –1.00 × 90	VA 20/30+ (6/9)
	OS: +3.25 –1.25 × 90	VA 20/25– (6/7.5–)
Phoria:	N/E	N/E
Base-in vergences:	N/E	N/E
Base-out vergences:	N/E	N/E
Accom. Amplitude:	0.25 each eye	
Neg. Rel. Accom.:	N/E	
Pos. Rel. Accom.:	N/E	
Fused X-Cyl.:	+2.50 VA 20/25– each eye	
Stereo:	N/E	

Assessment

Nuclear cataracts OU verified. Lens prescription accurate.

Plan

1. Educate AE regarding cataracts, cataract surgery, dietary therapy.
2. Discuss the advantages of the new glasses at both distance and near *and their limitations.*

AE's return several weeks after receiving her glasses with a complaint of poor vision suggests that she is not prepared for the limitations of her new glasses imposed by the cataracts. Discussion has to carefully describe the situation, since the patient has great faith in her dietary counselor. However, if we are of a different opinion, the patient should understand our beliefs concerning the dietary effects on the cataracts. Since we had not seen the patient previously, we cannot measure any lens changes. If the patient persists in her opinion that the glasses, although better, are not good enough, consider referral to another practitioner for a second opinion. With AE's permission, we might like to talk to the nutritionist, too.

The reexamination shows that the prescription is appropriate. It becomes obvious during the discussion that these new glasses do not meet AE's expectations. In the past, each lens change resulted in a more satisfactory level of corrected vision. The current situation may have been compounded by the fact that her dietary counselor apparently gave her the impression that the cataracts will be or are getting better.

It is possible that this disappointment with the new glasses could have been averted by the application of **clinical pearl 16**, "Exert care in advising what benefit the patient can expect with the new correction." In these situations, use trial lenses to demonstrate to the patient how he or she will see with the new glasses and compare with the old, indicating that this is the best-corrected vision possible. This could flow into a discussion of her cataracts and our professional opinion concerning her options.

Patient AF was an atypical illustration of **clinical pearl 5**, "Be careful about reducing the plus power at near with a presbyopic patient." Pertinent findings from the recheck visit follow.

Subjective

Case History, Including Signs, Symptoms, and Visual Needs
AF is a 43-year-old man who originally presented with difficulties seeing at near with his single-vision glasses, which he wore all of the time. He was prescribed a new bifocal correction for

constant wear. He returns 3 weeks later, saying that he sees better at near when he removes his old glasses than when he looks through the new bifocal segments.

New glasses,

OD: –2.00 DS/+1.00 add
OS: –2.00 DS/+1.00 add

Previous glasses,

OD: –2.00 DS
OS: –2.00 DS

Clinical Measures

		At 20 ft (6 m)	*At 16 in. (40 cm)*
VA (with bifocal prescription):	OD:	20/20 (6/6)	20/20 (6/6)
	OS:	20/20 (6/6)	20/20 (6/6)
Cover Test:		N/E	N/E
N.P.C.:		N/E	
Retinoscopy/	OD:	–2.00 DS	
Autorefractor:	OS:	–2.00 DS	
Subjective:	OD:	–2.00 DS	VA 20/20 (6/6)
	OS:	–2.00 DS	VA 20/20 (6/6)
Phoria:		3 eso	Ortho
Base-in vergences:		X/11/16	12/14/7
Base-out vergences:		N/E	X/14/8
Accom. Amplitude:		4.0	
Neg. Rel. Accom.:		N/E	
Pos. Rel. Accom.:		N/E	
Fused X-Cyl.:		+1.00 resulting in 20/20 (6/6) and 1 exop at 16 in. (40 cm)	
Stereo:		N/E	
Phoria through +2.00 Tentative Addition:		5 exop	

Assessment

The prescription (including an add for near) is confirmed.

Plan

1. New bifocal correction
   OD: –2.00 DS/+2.00 add
   OS: –2.00 DS/+2.00 add
2. Or, suggest that AF remove his distance prescription for reading and close work. The prescription with the +1.00 add is consistent with the clinical findings and more typical for a first bifocal but is unsuccessful because it defies **clinical pearl 5A**, "Be cautious about reducing the net plus power at near with a presbyopic patient." The result of the initial examination was to reduce the plus power at near from plano to –1.00 (–2.00 at distance with a +1.00 add results in –1.00 at near, and when he removes his glasses, –2.00 DS, so he sees through plano with the bonus of a full field of view). The original doctor did not note whether AF removes his glasses for near work and probably would do so when comparing his new glasses with his previous ones. When it becomes apparent that he compares the clarity at near with no glasses (using his myopia), the choices become more obvious. In either case, it is useful to measure or estimate the phoria at near with the plano prescription or, at the very least, ascertain whether AF is symptomatic when he reads without glasses.
3. This patient should have an explanation of presbyopia and its implications with his refractive state now and in the future.

Sometimes we go against one of our clinical pearls or at least replace it with another. This is exemplified by patient AG. The results of the recheck visit follow.

Subjective

Case History, Including Signs, Symptoms, and Visual Needs
AG, a 59-year-old woman, returns to the clinic after having received new glasses 2 weeks ago. She reports that, with her new glasses, she is seeing well at distance but has to hold reading matter closer than her preferred 20 in. (50 cm).

Lensometry

OD: −1.50 −0.50 × 90/+2.25 add

OS: −0.75 −1.25 × 90/+2.25 add

Objective

Ocular Health Assessment

N/E

Clinical Measures

		At 20 ft (6 m)	*At 16 in. (40 cm)*
VA (with	OD:	20/20 (6/6)	20/20 (6/6)
prescription):	OS:	20/20− (6/6−)	20/20− (6/6−)
Cover Test:		N/E	N/E
N.P.C.:		N/E	
Retinoscopy/	OD:	−1.50 −0.50 × 90	
Autorefractor:	OS:	−1.00 −1.00 × 80	
Subjective:	OD:	−1.50 −0.50 × 90	VA 20/20 (6/6)
	OS:	−1.00 −1.00 × 80	VA 20/20 (6/6)
Phoria:		N/E	N/E
Base-in vergences:		N/E	N/E
Base-out vergences:		N/E	N/E
Accom. Amplitude:		N/E	
Neg Rel. Accom.:		N/E	
Pos. Rel. Accom.:		N/E	
Fused X-Cyl.:		(At preferred working distance) +1.75 VA 20/20 (6/6) in each eye at 20 in. (50 cm)	
Stereo:		N/E	

Assessment

The new near prescription is too strong for her preferred working distance.

Plan

Place the tentative prescription in a trial frame. Since no space distortion is reported and vision is clear at desired reading distance, reorder new glasses as follows:

OD: −1.50 −0.50 × 90 / +1.75 add
OS: −1.00 −1.00 × 80 / +1.75 add

The tentative prescription at near should be carefully demonstrated to AG with an explanation that, if she holds reading matter closer, they will be less effective, reminding her why she returned. They might be described to her as "20 in. (50 cm) glasses."

The pearl we defy with AG is **clinical pearl 5**, "Be careful about reducing plus at near with a presbyopic patient," although she had only 2 weeks with the higher add. This illustrates that we can ignore some of these rules some of the time—with caution. A vital piece of information is missing from AG's original record chart: her preferred near working distance. Not everyone needs or prefers to function at 16 in. (40 cm).

Patient AH's return may or may not have been averted. The results of the original and second visit are presented. The initial visit's findings follow.

Subjective

Case History, Including Signs, Symptoms, and Visual Needs

AH is an 89-year-old man with cataract OD. He had cataract surgery OS 10 years ago, aphakic in that left eye. He is not happy with vision in either eye, particularly the "operated eye," which he notes is quite bad when he covers the OD. He wonders why he bothered to have the operation since he uses the OD almost exclusively. AH also feels self-conscious that his glasses look strange. The OD is slowly getting worse. He drives (primarily during daylight hours) and reads at 16 in. (40 cm). Reading is "OK" but that, too, "could be better." He noticed that when he holds things very close he can read better without glasses than with them, but he does not like holding the newspaper that close. He prefers two pair of glasses to bifocals.

Lensometry
OD: −4.50 DS
OS: +7.50 DS
OU: +2.50 add, single vision distance and near

Objective

Ocular Health Assessment

Cortical lens changes OD, aphakia OS (no implant). Everything else is unremarkable.

Clinical Measures

	At 20 ft (6 m)	At 16 in. (40 cm)
VA (with prescription):	OD: 20/25 –2 (6/7.5 –2)	20/30 (6/9)
	OS: 20/200 (6/60)	20/200 (6/60)
Cover Test:	Ortho	Sl exop
N.P.C.:	Suppression of OS	
Retinoscopy/ Autorefractor:	OD: –4.25 DS	
	OS: +9.25 –0.75 × 100	
Subjectjve:	OD: –4.25 DS	VA 20/25 (6/7.5)
	OS: +9.25 –0.75 × 100	VA 20/40 (6/12)
Phoria:	Suppression of OS at all distances	
Base-in vergences:	N/E	N/E
Base-out vergences:	N/E	N/E
Accom. Amplitude:	N/E	
Neg. Rel. Accom.:	N/E	
Pos. Rel. Accom.:	N/E	
Fused X-Cyl.:	No fusion, monoc. X-cyl +2.75 add	
Stereo:	Suppression of OS	

Assessment

Incipient cortical cataract and myopia OD, aphakia OS.

Plan

1. Prescribe slight lens change OD.
2. Prescribe new lens OS, which allows him the "peace of mind" that he can achieve better vision in the eye that had the surgery. AH is told that, when he covers the OD, he will see better with his OS than with the previous prescription.
3. Explain to him how he does not use both eyes together and what options exist if the OD continues to deteriorate.
4. Review what is a cataract and its progression.

5. Discuss a contact lens option, rejected by the patient. Prescription:
   OD: –4.25   VA 20/25– (6/7.5–)
   OS: +9.50 –0.75 × 100   VA 20/40+ (6/12+)
   OU: +2.75 add, single vision distance and near
6. AH should be told why his glasses "look strange," and they cannot be altered with a single pair of glasses that would provide him with best vision.

AH returned 2 weeks after receiving his glasses.

Subjective

Case History, Including Signs, Symptoms, and Visual Needs

At this visit, AH reports diplopia some of the time when he wears the distance glasses. He can eliminate this by covering one eye. He says that he sees better with these glasses in his OS than with his old glasses. However, when he tries his old glasses, he does not see double.

Lensometry verified that the glasses were fabricated as ordered. Testing revealed the following.

Objective

Ocular Health Assessment
N/E

Clinical Measures

Refraction (and VA): The same as when prescribed at previous visit
Cover Test: Intermittent left exotropia
The OS was suppressed with all binocular tests performed during the examination.

Assessment

Intermittent left exotropia with infrequent, but bothersome, diplopia with new prescription, although it is very difficult to clinically elicit binocularity as evidenced by the test results. For some reason, the patient persists in defying the odds.

Plan

Discourage binocularity by the prescribing of a cosmetically balanced lens OS. Prescribe

OD: −4.25 DS
OS: −2.00 DS (balance lens)
OU: +2.75 add, single vision distance and near

AH needs to justify in his own mind having had the surgery in the OS. The previous doctor probably felt that she could satisfy this need at no risk, since there apparently was no evidence of any binocular function during the examination visit. However, at that time, it would have been prudent to use trial lenses. When the acuity of the left eye improved, this barrier to binocularity was removed and diplopia resulted. The unequal size differences of the two retinal images would inhibit fusion but did not discourage binocularity. This situation verifies the utilization of **clinical pearl 15**, "The previous doctor may be wiser than initially realized," as well as **clinical pearl 4**, "Use trial lenses with every significant lens change."

AH requires careful education. He must understand that, if necessary, the OS is capable of better vision than he experienced when he entered with his previous glasses and the OD probably not as well as in the past because of the cataract progression. This new prescription should eliminate the diplopia and give him spectacles that are cosmetically "normal."

He also needs to be informed about the possibility of the OD needing surgery in the future and the postsurgical vision implications. AH's aphakic OS is an unusual occurrence these days and may present an optical dilemma in the future if surgery with the OD is contemplated with intraocular lenses.

One can only guess whether this diplopia would have been elicited with trial lenses. The examiner had good reason to assume that AH would suppress the OS.

AH should be told that, for very precise near detail, he can remove his glasses and use his OD alone at about 10 in. (25 cm) and the reasons why this is so. He should be assured that he will not ruin his eyes by holding near-seeing matter at this close distance.

Another variation of this was AI. At her initial visit the following was found.

Subjective

Case History, Including Signs, Symptoms, and Visual Needs

AI is a 39-year-old homemaker, who reads at 16 in. (40 cm). She reports no special visual needs or problems, presenting for a routine eye exam. She reports seeing well. Her ocular history is unremarkable, and other than taking thyroid medication, she enjoys good health. Her present prescription is 4 years old.

Lensometry
OD: –3.50 DS
OS: –3.25 DS

Objective

Ocular Health Assessment
No evidence of ocular or systemic pathology.

Clinical Measures

	At 20 ft (6 m)	At 16 in. (40 cm)
VA (previous	OD: 20/40+ (6/12+)	20/20 (6/6)
prescription):	OS: 20/20 –2 (6/6 –2)	20/20 (6/6)
Cover Test:	Ortho	
N.P.C.:	To the nose	
Retinoscopy/	OD: –4.25 DS	
Autorefractor:	OS: –3.50 DS	
Subjective:	OD: –4.25 DS	VA 20/20 (6/6)
	OS: –3.50 DS	VA 20/20 (6/6)
Phoria (through subj.)	2 esop	Ortho
Base-in vergences:	X/8/5	N/E
Base-out vergences:	N/E	N/E
Accom. Amplitude:	4.50	
Neg. Rel. Accom.:	+1.50 (through +0.75 tentative add)	
Pos. Rel. Accom.:	–1.50	
Fused X-Cyl.:	+0.75	
Stereo:	N/E	

Assessment

Eyes healthy, myopia, early presbyopia(?).

Plan

1. New lenses ordered:
   OD: –4.00 DS
   OS: –3.50 DS
   OU: +0.75 add, single-vision lenses for distance and near
   Discuss the possibility of a bifocal form. AI prefers single-vision lenses.
2. Instruct AI to return in 2 years.
3. Educate AI concerning presbyopia.

AI returns 4 weeks later, reporting pain in her eyes with the new glasses. She does not use the two new pairs but prefers her old glasses, which she feels are good for all seeing needs. The result of the recheck visit is

OD: –3.50 DS
OS: –3.25 DS

for all visual needs.

AI presents the problem of the slightly undercorrected myope on the cusp of presbyopia. If she had an entering complaint of poor distance vision, perhaps she would have accepted the original doctor's approach, particularly if it were carefully discussed and illustrated. AI remains a problem waiting to happen, as she will become more presbyopic, so it is necessary to prepare her for this eventuality. The degree of undercorrection will extend the delay of clinical presbyopia.

AI is somewhat similar to patient AA, except that AA required improved acuity because she drives a bus and removes her distance correction when she reads.

Although our dissatisfied patient clinic did not often see contact lens patients, we experienced a parallel situation with AJ, who at age 39 decided to use contact lenses. The contact lens doctor, wishing to demonstrate how well she was capable of seeing and possibly ignoring the accommodative differences with contact lenses, also created a patient who is clinically presbyopic, causing unhappiness. Becoming immersed in this situation was easier than extricating oneself. AJ likes her new, improved vision with the contact lenses but not the newly observed diminished near-vision side effects. One "solution" was to encourage her to wear the contact lenses and explain the reasons for, then prescribe, a near correction to be worn with the contact lenses. Other approaches would be bifocal contact lenses or monovision. Apparently, as a result of this discussion, the patient understands the situation and its dilemmas. (It should have been part of the contact lens patient management.) AJ also is advised that, if she chooses to, she can continue to wear her old spectacle correction at work, since AJ uses a computer at work and the glasses are fine for this task. However, since she prefers her contact lenses, the following is prescribed:

OU: +0.75 DS (to be worn over the contacts, for near only)

The excellent distance vision created by the contacts figuratively released the genie from the bottle, to which it cannot be returned. Apparently, she is satisfied with her options.

Patient AK had a different complaint with his 1-month-old glasses.

Subjective

Case History, Including Signs, Symptoms, and Visual Needs
AK is a 72-year-old retiree who reports that he sees relatively well at distance with his glasses, although he uses his right eye almost exclusively. His problems are mainly at near, where his best clarity in the right eye is at approximately 14 in. (36 cm) and the best vision at near with his left eye is at 9 in. (23 cm). He personally verifies this by covering one eye and then the other. The difference in acuity at distance does not seem to bother him. He says that the doctor told him, several years ago, that he had an "aging problem in his left eye," which was verified at the last visit.

Lensometry

OD: +2.50 −0.75 × 90 / +2.50 add
OS: +1.75 −0.50 × 90 / +4.00 add

Objective

Ocular Health Assessment

Confirmed age-related macular degeneration (ARMD) OS.

Clinical Measures

		At 20 ft (6 m)	At 16 in. (40 cm)
VA (with	OD:	20/20 (6/6)	20/20 (6/6)
prescription):	OS:	20/80 (6/24)	20/80 (6/24)
Cover Test:		N/E	N/E

Patient measures 20/50 (6/15) at 10 in. (25 cm) with OS = focal distance of +4.00 DS.

N.P.C.:		N/E	
Retinoscopy/	OD:	+2.50 −0.75 × 90	
Autorefractor:	OS:	+2.00 −0.50 × 90	
Subjective:	OD:	+2.50 −0.75 × 90	VA 20/20− (6/6−)
	OS:	+1.75 −0.50 × 90	VA 20/80 (6/24)
Phoria:		N/E	N/E
Base-in vergences:		N/E	N/E
Base-out vergences:		N/E	N/E
Accom. Amplitude:		0.50 each eye	
Neg. Rel. Accom.:		N/E	
Pos. Rel. Accom.:		N/E	
Fused X-Cyl.:		+2.50	
Stereo:		N/E	
Near Ranges,	OD:	13–16 in.	VA 20/20 (6/6)
Previous Prescription:		(33–40 cm) with 2.50 add	
	OS:	9–10 in. (23–25 cm) with +4.00 add	VA 20/50 (6/15)

Near range with +2.50 add OS 13–16 in. (33–40 cm) 20/80 (6/24) VA

Assessment

Unequal adds causing unequal near ranges. Compound hyperopic astigmia OU. Reduced acuity OS due to ARMD.

Plan
1. Prescribe a new add for the OS to equalize near ranges:
   OD: +2.50 –0.75 × 90/+2.50 add
   OS: +1.75 –0.50 × 90/+2.50 add
2. Educate AK concerning ARMD and the spectacle correction.

AK's situation teaches us an important lesson. Although the use of the +4.00 add OS would be consistent with the needs of a patient having 20/80 acuity, it disturbs the near focal balance and bothers the patient. This is consistent with **clinical pearl 22**, "Balanced accommodative focus levels help to ensure happy patients." This patient does not meet the definition of a low-vision patient, since his right eye has good correctable acuity. When the two eyes are not capable of equal vision and the patient is capable of binocular fusion with no central suppression, it is more comfortable to the patient visually to have equal distances of clarity rather than best possible clarity at unequal distances. Accommodative balance is highly desirable at both distance and near. The +2.50 add over the left eye would produce a similar range although with lowered acuity when compared to the right eye.

AL is someone else's patient. This patient's problem may have been caused by an overzealous practitioner. The findings are as follows.

Subjective

Case History, Including Signs, Symptoms, and Visual Needs
AL is a 68-year-old man who is unhappy with the horizontal bifocal line on his left lens. He received the glasses 1 month ago and never had this type of lens before. He was told by the doctor that cataracts have caused his two eyes to be different, requiring a special grinding to encourage him to read with both his eyes. He has no other significant history.

Lensometry

OD: +4.00 DS/+2.50 add
OS: +1.25 DS/+2.50 add = 2 prism diopters base up
OU: Flat-top 25-mm bifocals with slab-off OS.

Objective

Ocular Health Assessment

Since we had not seen this patient before nor had access to previous records, all appropriate tests were performed. Other than nuclear cataracts, OU, OS more than OD, his eyes are healthy.

Clinical Measures

		At 20 ft (6 m)	*At 16 in. (40 cm)*
VA (with	OD:	20/20– (6/6–)	20/20 (6/6)
prescription):	OS:	20/40 (6/12)	20/40 (6/12)
Cover Test:		Exoph	LX(T)′
N.P.C.:		Suppression of OS	
Retinoscopy/	OD:	+4.00 DS	
Autorefractor:	OS:	+1.00 DS	
Subjective:	OD:	+4.00 DS	VA 20/20– (6/6–)
	OS:	+1.25 DS	VA 20/40 (6/12)
Phoria:		10 exop	Supp OS
Base-in vergences:		N/E	N/E
Base-out vergences:		X/18/8	Supp OS
Accom. Amplitude:		0.50 each eye	
Neg. Rel. Accom.:		N/E	
Pos. Rel. Accom.:		N/E	
Fused X-Cyl.:		N/E	
Plus Build-up:		+2.50 add	
Stereo:		Suppression of OS at near	

Assessment

Bilateral nuclear cataracts, OS more than OD; eyes otherwise healthy; hyperopia and presbyopia; exophoria at distance, left exotropia at near.

Plan

1. Monitor cataracts; patient not interested in surgical intervention at this time since he is seeing well.
2. Change OS prescription to eliminate the slab-off grinding:
   OD: +4.00 DS/+2.50 add
   OS: +1.25 DS/+2.50 add
3. Discuss the ocular reasons for the elimination of the slab-off grinding. Fortunately, this coincides with his concerns relating to the cosmetic appearance of his glasses.

AL receives no appreciable benefit from the slab-off prism, since he suppresses the left eye at near and the horizontal line cosmetically bothers him. Prior to prescribing a slab-off prism, the doctor must have been certain that the vertical prism would enhance binocularly at near. Anisometropia at near, by itself, is insufficient justification to prescribe slab-off prism.

Patient AM's situation is related to his systemic medication.

Subjective

Case History, Including Signs, Symptoms, and Visual Needs

AM, a 34-year-old stock clerk, originally enters with complaints more typical of presbyopia. He says that he is having difficulty seeing at near and "his arms are too short too see small print clearly," although it improves when he moves reading matter away. This problem seems to have started approximately 1 year ago. He never wore glasses or had a "real" eye examination, since his vision was "always 20/20." He has been having health problems over the past year, taking Bentyl for his irritated bowel and, more recently, erythromycin for a sore throat, which is improving. There are no other significant problems in his or his family's health history. AM reads at 16 in. (40 cm); his computer terminal is at 25 in. (64 cm); he watches television and drives an automobile. The results of the original examination are as follows.

Objective

Ocular Health Assessment

Reviewing the possible ocular side effects of Bentyl and erythromycin indicates that, while erythromycin has few, Bentyl has several. The tests reveal no significant mydriasis or increased intraocular pressure (16 mm Hg Goldmann).

Clinical Measures

	At 20 ft (6 m)	*At 16 in. (40 cm)*
VA (no prescription):	OD: 20/20 (6/6)	20/20– (6/6–)
	OS: 20/20 (6/6)	20/20– (6/6–)
Cover Test:	Ortho (horiz and vert)	Exop
N.P.C.:	3 in. (7.6 cm)/diplopia/4 in. (10 cm) recovery	
Retinoscopy/	OD: Plano –0.25 × 180	
Autorefractor:	OS: Plano –0.25 × 180	
Subjective:	OD: Plano –0.25 × 180	VA 20/20 (6/6)
	OS: Plano –0.25 × 180	VA 20/20 (6/6)
Phoria:	Ortho	2 exop
Base-in vergences:	N/E	N/E
Base-out vergences:	N/E	X/12/8
Accom. Amplitude:	3.00 each eye	
Neg. Rel. Accom.:	2.25	
Pos. Rel. Accom.:	1.00	
Fused X-Cyl.:	+1.50, 9 exop with this tentative add	
Stereo:	N/E	

Assessment

AM's examination reveals an accommodative insufficiency that would be more typical of a patient approximately 10 years older. The onset of these near problems appears to coincide with his taking Bentyl. The literature indicates that Bentyl can affect the accommodative mechanism, and it appears that this may be a cause of the apparent early presbyopia.

Plan

It is prudent when a patient is taking medications to research whether the drugs have ocular side effects. In that event, as with Bentyl, this would explain some of the examination results and the following was prescribed:

OU: +0.50 DS/+0.75 add *for computer and reading only*

AM returns 1 month later, stating that the glasses, while apparently "OK" at first, appear unnecessary recently. He describes his vision being clear for near work, but with prolonged reading, he has a pulling sensation. He is doing much better physically, and his physician has taken him off all medications. The results of the dissatisfied patient visit show that he now requires no spectacle correction. His amplitude of accommodation is 6.00 diopters (push-up) and other findings, including the positive relative accommodation, are consistent with expected values. The reexam clinician surmises that the pulling sensation may result from attempting to compensate for the convergence insufficiency that surfaces with the added plus power prescribed but no longer needed for near. The retesting of findings indicated that AM's AC/A ratio remains as before. As a result, during this visit, we explain to AM that, in the future, as his physiological accommodative levels diminish, the lens correction necessary may again cause him to experience this pulling sensation with prolonged close work. He is advised to return again in 2 years and is told that, at that time, it might be desirable to consider vision therapy to prevent the near discomfort that may accompany glasses in the future.

With dissatisfied patients, we always consider whether the second visit could have been prevented. The original doctor was functioning appropriately by investigating the ocular side effects of the patient's medication. The proximity of the use of Bentyl and AM's awareness of the symptoms show the wisdom of the doctor to investigate all the effects of this drug. AM did not demonstrate the other possible side effects of the drug and the original prescription was to compensate for the diminished accommodative levels.

Exercising the ability to second-guess the original doctor, it was felt that two separate issues might have been addressed during the first visit. The most important was that, after learning the possible effects of the drug Bentyl, the examiner should have contacted AM's physician to learn whether this medication was likely for long- or short-term use. If the patient is to discontinue the drug shortly, it is of dubious value to prescribe spectacles for its effects. If it will be a long-term therapy, lenses to compensate could be prescribed; however, the patient and his physician should be aware that future changes in the drug therapy might require changes in the spectacle lenses.

The other issue was the apparent oversight by the original examiner to indicate to the patient that there was a potential convergence problem. This could have been done in a manner that would inform the patient without necessarily suggesting the symptoms. The original doctor failed to advise the patient that he might experience symptoms with prolonged close work, as suggested by the near phoria findings through the additional plus power and his compensating ranges.

Damage Control with the Dissatisfied Patient

The cases reviewed here represent the primary aspect of the damage control needed with the dissatisfied patient. Be pleased when the patient gives you the opportunity to rectify the situation, and this should be apparent in your behavior. (The patient will sense if you are annoyed and this will mitigate against a solution.) Some of the rules that apply to virtually all of these patients are these:

1. Ask what brings the patient in and listen to his or her responses. Patients often tell you what they perceive is wrong, and more important, they may offer a solution. A frequent example is the patient who says he sees better if he changes how the glasses sit on his face to alter the effective power of the lenses. The questioning should be phrased in language and tone that does not suggest anything other than your desire to help.

2. After the patient lists the problems a good response is, "I can understand your wanting to return. I would feel the same way." Whether or not patients wish to be confrontational, you are giving them no reason to be hostile and are appearing sensitive to their immediate needs. You should care and give that impression. If the doctor makes closure prematurely, either by prejudging the reliability of the patient or the feasibility of another approach, there is less likelihood of resolution.

3. Retest all findings, including lensometry, that are pertinent to resolving the new presenting problems. Most of the situations we have observed are spectacle-related problems. In the event, after some retesting, you find no need to change anything, the patients will not feel that you "blew them off." In this situation, the patients need to be told that your findings indicate that the original prescription was appropriate. Be certain that the glasses fit as they should and the patient understands when to use them. At times, a different utilization of the same prescription neutralizes the problem.

4. If a change is necessary, recommend it. Failure to make changes should be based on evidence, not stubbornness. Sometimes, a small change brings patient satisfaction. In this situation the clinician might consider contradicting **clinical pearl 9**, which states, "In general, a lens change of less than 0.50 diopters seldom diminishes subjective symptoms." Whether it is the small change, your willingness to listen and make a modest change, or employing a placebo, we have observed success in this approach.

5. Fully discuss why the patient perceives a problem and how you suggest rectifying it. If the problem resulted from a different interpretation of data, tell the patient. Patients are becoming more sophisticated and understand that doctoring requires judgments. It often is useful to assure the patients that wearing the previous prescription would not have caused damage to their eyes. You might choose to use other examples familiar to them in the discussion. Patients understand that treatment sometimes comes with side effects. The best preventative is to discuss some of these possibilities at

dispensing; **see clinical pearl 18**, "Remind patients that they may have to adapt to their new glasses."

6. As mentioned earlier, we find that most of the returning patients have problems that can be resolved in the dispensary. The dispensary should verify that the glasses are *exactly* as ordered and fit properly. A well-fitted, properly fabricated spectacle is a wonderfully successful therapeutic device.

7. Some patients need to be advised to give the new glasses a reasonable time for their adaptation. We find that 2 weeks is a reasonable period to allow for this, provided the patient wears them as prescribed.

8. In spite of your best efforts, some patients have problems you are unable to solve. It is necessary for you to express this to them, indicating that you want to consult with colleagues and read the literature; if you have anything to discuss with them, you will contact them. Patients can be comforted that advances in health care are continuous and you will be alert to anything that may benefit them. If the symptoms remain disturbing—and these are incredibly rare—offer to refer them to another practitioner or facility. A subset among these are those patients who require a re-examination every time they receive care. Many of these patients need frequent reassurance and counseling about their eyes and have entered your care with an agenda, hidden or otherwise, that was not resolved in their minds.

9. Encourage patients to feel comfortable contacting your office if they ever have any questions relating to their eyes or their glasses. This keeps the door open for you to remain their doctor. Some patients need to be assured that they are not annoying you.

In Summary,

1. Reevaluate the history using open-ended questions that allow the patient to talk.
2. Take and recheck pertinent findings, particularly those relating to lens fabrication.

3. Reanalyze the patient's needs, problems, treatment options, and the like.
4. If no change is necessary, be certain the patient understands the utilization as well as the limitations of the glasses, citing as many clinical pearls as appropriate.
5. If another lens prescription is necessary, recheck and duplicate all the parameters of all appropriate glasses and their adjustment on the face.

Reference

1. Glasses. *Consumer Reports.* July 1997;62(7):10–15.

Index

Page references followed by "t" denote tables; "f" denote figures.